100 Questions & Answers About Your Digestive Health:
A Lahey Clinic Guide

Edited by

Andrew S. Warner, MD

Chairman
Department of Gastroenterology
Lahey Clinic
Burlington, MA

D0770513

JONES AND BARTLETT PUBLISHERS
Sudbury, Massachusetts
BOSTON   TORONTO   LONDON   SINGAPORE

World Headquarters
Jones and Bartlett Publishers
40 Tall Pine Drive
Sudbury, MA 01776
978-443-5000
info@jbpub.com
www.jbpub.com

Jones and Bartlett Publishers
Canada
6339 Ormindale Way
Mississauga, Ontario L5V 1J2
Canada

Jones and Bartlett Publishers
International
Barb House, Barb Mews
London W6 7PA
United Kingdom

Jones and Bartlett's books and products are available through most bookstores and online booksellers. To contact Jones and Bartlett Publishers directly, call 800-832-0034, fax 978-443-8000, or visit our website, www.jbpub.com.

Substantial discounts on bulk quantities of Jones and Bartlett's publications are available to corporations, professional associations, and other qualified organizations. For details and specific discount information, contact the special sales department at Jones and Bartlett via the above contact information or send an email to specialsales@jbpub.com.

The authors, editor, and publisher have made every effort to provide accurate information. However, they are not responsible for errors, omissions, or for any outcomes related to the use of the contents of this book and take no responsibility for the use of the products and procedures described. Treatments and side effects described in this book may not be applicable to all people; likewise, some people may require a dose or experience a side effect that is not described herein. Drugs and medical devices are discussed that may have limited availability controlled by the Food and Drug Administration (FDA) for use only in a research study or clinical trial. Research, clinical practice, and government regulations often change the accepted standard in this field. When consideration is being given to use of any drug in the clinical setting, the health care provider or reader is responsible for determining FDA status of the drug, reading the package insert, and reviewing prescribing information for the most up-to-date recommendations on dose, precautions, and contraindications, and determining the appropriate usage for the product. This is especially important in the case of drugs that are new or seldom used.

Production Credits

Executive Publisher: Christopher Davis
Editorial Assistant: Jessica Acox
Production Director: Amy Rose
Production Editor: Daniel Stone
Associate Marketing Manager: Ilana Goddess

Manufacturing Buyer: Therese Connell
Composition: Jason Miranda/Spoke & Wheel
Cover Design: Jonathan Ayotte
Printing and Binding: Malloy, Inc.
Cover Printing: Malloy, Inc.

Cover Credits:
[Top Left] © Carsten Reisinger/ShutterStock, Inc.; [Top Right] © Andresr/ShutterStock, Inc.;
[Bottom] © LE Media/ShutterStock, Inc.

Library of Congress Cataloging-in-Publication Data
Warner, Andrew S.
   100 questions & answers about your digestive health / Andrew S. Warner.
      p. cm.
   Includes bibliographical references and index.
   ISBN-13: 978-0-7637-5327-6
   ISBN-10: 0-7637-5327-0
   1. Digestive organs--Diseases--Popular works. 2. Digestion--Popular
works. I. Title. II. Title: 100 questions and answers about your digestive
health. III. Title: One hundred questions & answers about your digestive
health.
   RC806.W37 2009
   616.3--dc22
                                          2008004038
6048
Printed in the United States of America
12 11 10 09 08   10 9 8 7 6 5 4 3 2 1

Contents

Contributors

Amy E. Barto, MD, was born and raised in Cheshire, Connecticut. She graduated from Dartmouth College in 1995 and attended the University of Connecticut Medical School. She completed her residency in internal medicine and fellowship in gastroenterology at the Lahey Clinic. She is currently a member of the Department of Gastroenterology at Lahey Clinic specializing in inflammatory bowel disease. She is also an Assistant Clinical Professor of Medicine at Tufts University School of Medicine.

Stephen C. Fabry, MD, is a senior staff physician at Lahey Clinic in Massachusetts. He specializes in the treatment of patients with liver disease including hepatitis C and evaluation for liver transplantation. Dr. Fabry graduated from New York University School of Medicine where he was elected to the Alpha Omega Alpha Honor Medical Society. He completed his medical residency at Beth Israel.

Eric D. Goldberg, MD, is a Senior Staff Physician at Lahey Clinic in Burlington, Massachusetts. Dr. Goldberg graduated from Hahnemann Medical College. He completed his medical residency at University of Massachusetts Medical Center in Worcester, Massachusetts and his gastroenterology fellowship at Lahey Clinic in Burlington, Massachusetts. Dr. Goldberg completed his fellowship in Transplant Hepatology at Beth Israel Deaconess Medical Center in Boston, Massachusetts and Lahey Clinic. In addition to his expertise in liver disease, he has an interest in general gastrointestinal disorders.

Stephen J. Heller, MD, is a senior staff physician and director of endoscopy at the Lahey Clinic. Dr. Heller did his undergraduate studies at Yale University and received his medical degree from the Columbia University College of Physicians and Surgeons. He completed his residency in internal medicine at Stanford University Hospital and fellowship in gastroenterology at the Brigham and Women's Hospital, Harvard Medical School, with additional training in advanced endoscopic procedures at the Wellesley Hospital, University of Toronto. Dr. Heller has served as the fellowship training director in gastroenterology at the Lahey Clinic and has been a member of the admissions committee of Tufts University School of Medicine. Dr. Heller's clinical and research interests include diagnosis and management of disorders of the pancreas, gallbladder and biliary system, endoscopic palliation of gastrointestinal malignancy, and medical education.

Ann Marie Joyce, MD, is the Director of Endoscopic Ultrasound and Senior Staff Gastroenterologist at the Lahey Clinic in Burlington, Massachusetts. Dr. Joyce completed her internal medicine residency and gastroenterology fellowship at Lahey Clinic. She then went to the University of Pennsylvania for a fourth year fellowship in advanced endoscopy. Her areas of interest include advanced endoscopy and gastrointestinal malignancies. She has authored many peer reviewed articles, chapters, and given lectures.

R. Anand Narasimhan, MD, is a Senior Staff Gastroenterologist at Lahey Clinic in Massachusetts. He was raised in Kingston, Rhode Island. After earning his medical degree from the University of Vermont, he completed an internal medicine residency at Mayo Clinic in Rochester, Minnesota. He currently practices general gastroenterology. Dr. Narasimhan is an Assistant Clinical Professor of Medicine at Tufts University School of Medicine.

Stephen F. Nezhad, MD, is currently a staff physician in Gastroenterology at Lahey Clinic Northshore in Peabody, Massachusetts. He grew up in Waterbury, Connecticut, the son of gastroenterologist. He was a biology major at Hamilton College in Clinton, New York and then attended the University of Connecticut School of Medicine. He completed his residency training in internal medicine at Maine Medical Center in Portland, Maine before completing his fellowship in gastroenterology at Lahey Clinic.

Kristen M. Robson, MD, is a senior staff gastroenterologist at Lahey Clinic and is an Assistant Clinical Professor of Medicine at Tufts University School of Medicine. She is co-director of the Gastrointestinal Motility Lab at Lahey Clinic and has authored several publications on the topics of gastrointestinal motility and functional bowel disease. She is an active member of the American College of Gastroenterology and the Massachusetts Medical Society. She completed her training in internal medicine and gastroenterology at Beth Israel Deaconess Medical Center and Harvard Medical School in Boston.

Introduction

If you've picked up this book, you are one of millions of people who are concerned about your health. You may want to learn more about your digestive system, have a question about a specific digestive disease or disorder, or simply be curious about what makes your body work. *100 Questions & Answers About Your Digestive Health: A Lahey Clinic Guide* is intended to be a patient-focused, practical guide to help you understand the digestive system and diseases of the gastrointestinal tract, liver, and pancreas. The questions are taken directly from the thousands we have been asked by real-life patients. The answers are a compilation of the latest scientific information along with our own experience in treating patients with digestive disorders. Written by Senior Staff Physicians in the Department of Gastroenterology at Lahey Clinic, this book also includes commentary by a number of patients with digestive problems. Filled with helpful hints and invaluable insights, this book will give you the tools to help navigate your way through the maze of medical jargon, confusing terminology, and seemingly complex digestive system.

In Part One, Dr. Eric Goldberg explores "the basics" of the digestive system. He describes the anatomy and function of the gastrointestinal tract, goes over what type of tests can be performed to evaluate the digestive system, and talks about many of the common symptoms that people can experience—diarrhea, constipation, bloating, and jaundice. He also reviews the effect that pregnancy can have on the digestive system, and discusses the most common digestive disorder—irritable bowel syndrome (IBS).

Part Two focuses on the upper gastrointestinal tract—the esophagus, stomach, and acid-related disorders. In this section, Dr. Stephen Nezhad discusses ulcers, heartburn, indigestion, problems swallowing, and *H. pylori* (*Helicobacter pylori*).

Part Three provides an in-depth review of the two most common types of inflammatory bowel diseases, Crohn's disease and ulcerative colitis. Written by Dr. Amy Barto, this section also goes over some less common types of intestinal inflammation including microscopic colitis, ischemic colitis, as well as diverticulosis.

Part Four highlights problems with malnutrition and malabsorption. Dr. Anand Narasimhan provides a detailed description of the causes of malnutrition and malabsorption, and discusses the effects these disorders have on our health. This section also reviews some of the more common malabsorptive syndromes, such as Celiac disease, lactose intolerance, specific nutrient and vitamin deficiencies, and also goes over common food allergies.

In the Part Five, Dr. Kristen Robson reviews the various intestinal infections, such as foodborne illnesses, travelers' diarrhea, and parasitic infections. Dr. Robson also discusses who is at risk for contracting an intestinal infection and ways to prevent getting such as infection.

Part Six is devoted to cancers of the digestive system. Dr. Ann Marie Joyce reviews cancer of the esophagus, stomach, liver, pancreas, and colon, and describes the differences between a traditional colonoscopy, virtual colonoscopy, and capsule endoscopy.

In Part Seven, Dr. Stephen Heller provides a detailed review of diseases of the pancreas and gallbladder, including acute and chronic pancreatitis, goes over how to tell if you have gallstones, and discusses how gallbladder disease is treated.

Part Eight is dedicated to the liver. In this last section, Dr. Stephen Fabry describes the function of the liver, what tests can be used to evaluate problems affecting the liver, and discusses many common liver diseases, including hepatitis A, B, and C, as well as fatty liver, hemochromatosis, cirrhosis, and liver transplantation.

100 Questions & Answers About Your Digestive Health: A Lahey Clinic Guide contains all the questions you wish you had asked your doctor and many that you never even thought to ask. For those interested in understanding more about digestive disorders, this book will provide you with the important information you need to know about your digestive health.

Andrew S. Warner, MD

PART ONE

The Basics

Eric D. Goldberg, MD

I often have diarrhea—what does this mean?

How would I know if I am bleeding from my intestines?

Can medications affect my digestive system?

More . . .

1. What is the digestive tract?

The digestive system [**Figure 1**] is a series of hollow organs joined in a long continuous tube—including the esophagus, stomach and intestines—beginning in the mouth and ending in the anus. This is called the alimentary canal. Other abdominal organs—including the **liver** and **pancreas**—play a part in digestion. The digestive tract is about 30 feet long.

The inside lining of these tubes is called **mucosa**. The mucosa contains glands, located in the mouth, **stomach**, and **small intestine**, produce juices or enzymes that aid in the digestion of food.

Liver

Solid organ of the alimentary tract involved in break-down of toxins and formation of proteins.

Pancreas

Oblong organ in the upper abdomen with two distinct functions: (1) Enzymes produced by the pancreas are critical for the digestion of food, and (2) Specialized cells in the pancreas called islet cells make insulin and glucagons, which control the levels of sugar in the bloodstream.

Mucosa

Inside lining of the intestinal tract.

Stomach

Organ that mixes and breaks down food particles.

Small intestine

The small bowel is made up of the duodenum, jejunum, and ileum. Anatomically it is found after the stomach and before the colon and is responsible for digestion and absorption of nutrients.

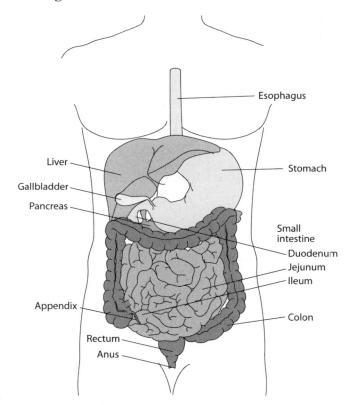

Figure 1 Digestive System. Copyright © 2007 Jones and Bartlett Publisers, Inc. (Warner, *100 Questions & Answers About Crohn's Disease.*)

Digestion begins in the mouth. **Salivary glands** located under the tongue begin the process of breaking down food. This is also aided by the action of chewing, which produces small particles of food that are easier to digest.

The action of swallowing then moves the food from the throat or **pharynx**, which then travels into the **esophagus**. Muscles within the walls of the esophagus push the food into the stomach. This action is known as **peristalsis**.

Once the food has made its way down the esophagus, it goes directly into the **stomach**. Stomach muscles mix and break down food with the help of digestive acid and enzymes, creating even smaller bits of food.

Food now leaving the stomach is pushed in to the small intestine. The small intestine is made up of three parts: **duodenum**, **jejunum**, and **ileum.** The small intestine is responsible for absorbing food and nutrients. Nutrients are absorbed in the small intestine by way of **villi,** which are small finger like projections that line the mucosa of the small intestine.

Though the **liver, gallbladder,** and **pancreas** are considered "solid organs" and not part of the alimentary canal, they are essential to digestive function.

The pancreas makes enzymes that work to digest proteins, fats, and carbohydrates. The liver produces **bile,** which is stored in the gallbladder. Bile is released from the gallbladder after eating to help absorb fat.

After food has not been digested, the remaining waste travels from the small intestine to the **large intestine.** By

Digestion begins in the mouth.

Salivary gland

Glands in the mouth that produce material that aid in the breakdown of food.

Pharynx

Structure in the throat that connects directly with the beginning of the intestinal tract or esophagus.

Esophagus

Tube that carries food from the mouth to the stomach.

Peristalsis

Movement of the muscles that line the intestinal tract.

Duodenum

The first part of the small intestine starting at the end of the stomach.

Gallbladder

Pouch connected to the bile ducts that stores bile which is released with eating to aid in digestion.

Colon

Large intestine that processes and stores waste.

Rectum

Last part of the colon where stool is stored before it leaves digestive tract.

Obstruction

A blockage; can be in any portion of the intestinal tract or bile ducts.

Perforation

A rupture or abnormal opening of the intestine.

Abscess

A walled-off collection of pus.

Upper GI series/ Upper GI series with small bowel follow through

A radiologic examination of the esophagus, stomach, duodenum, and small bowel.

Gastrointestinal tract

The digestive tube starting at the mouth and ending at the anus.

Stricture

A narrowed area of intestine usually due to scar tissue.

Fistula

A tunnel connecting two structures that are not normally connected.

the time food reaches the large intestine, all the essential nutrients have been absorbed by the small intestine. The large intestine works to remove water from the undigested material and form solid waste or stool.

The large intestine is made up of the **colon** and the **rectum**. The first part of the colon is the cecum. This is where the small intestine joins the large intestine. The last part of the colon joins the rectum where stool is stored until it leaves the digestive tract.

2. What type of tests can be done to evaluate the digestive system?

Abdominal X-ray: provides a picture of structures and organs in the abdomen and helpful in detecting a bowel **obstruction** or a **perforation**.

CT scan: uses X-rays to create a more detailed look inside the body. It is especially helpful in detecting an **abscess**, and also useful in evaluating for a bowel obstruction and perforation.

Upper GI series/Upper GI series with small bowel follow through: allows a close examination of the esophagus, stomach, duodenum, and small bowel by having the patient drink a thick, white liquid shake of barium, and then taking X-rays as it goes through the **gastrointestinal tract**. This is an excellent test to detect **strictures, fistulas**, and **inflammation** in the stomach and small bowel.

Barium enema: allows a close examination of the rectum and colon by instilling barium through the rectum and taking X-rays as it goes through the colon. This is an excellent test to detect strictures, inflammation, and fistulas in the colon.

Enteroclysis: provides a detailed examination of the small **bowel** by passing a small tube through the nose, into the stomach, and out into the duodenum. Barium is then instilled through the tube and directly into the small bowel. This is an excellent test to detect small abnormalities in the small intestine that may not have been seen on small bowel follow through.

Ultrasound: uses sound waves to examine abdominal and pelvic organs. It is commonly used to look for **gallstones** and obstruction of the **bile duct**.

MRI: uses a magnetic field to create a detailed picture of the structures and organ in the abdomen and pelvis. This is especially helpful in detecting abdominal and pelvic abscesses; it can also be used to evaluate the bile duct and pancreatic duct.

Virtual colonoscopy: a CT scan of the colon. This radiologic examination is still in early development but shows promise as a method to detect colonic abnormalities

Upper endoscopy: usually performed under **sedation**, a small, thin, flexible, lighted tube with a camera on the end is passed through the mouth into the esophagus, stomach, and duodenum. This is an excellent test to detect inflammation and strictures in the upper GI tract, and allows for a **biopsy** to be taken.

Colonoscopy: usually performed under sedation, a small, thin, flexible lighted tube with a camera on the end is passed through the rectum into the colon and, at times, the ileum. This is an excellent test to detect inflammation and strictures in the rectum, colon, and ileum, and allows for a biopsy to be taken.

Enteroclysis
A radiologic examination that provides a detailed examination of the small bowel.

Bowel
Term used for both the large and small intestines.

Ultrasound
Noninvasive form of X-ray imaging using sound waves.

Gallstones
Particles ranging in size from fine specks to firm concretions one inch in diameter.

Bile duct
Tube connecting the liver and small intestine.

MRI
A type of X-ray exam which uses magnetic energy.

Virtual colonoscopy
CT scan of the colon.

Upper endoscopy (EGD)
An examination in which a flexible lighted tube with a camera on the end is inserted through the mouth into the esophagus, stomach, and duodenum.

Colonoscopy
An instrument inserted into the rectum to examine the colon.

Sigmoidoscopy

This procedure is basically a "short" colonoscopy and is used to examine the rectum and left colon.

Proctoscopy

A procedure in which a rigid, straight, lighted tube is used to examine the rectum; usually on a special tilt table that positions the patient with the head down and butt up.

Anoscopy

A procedure in which a rigid, short, straight, lighted tube is used to examine the anal canal; usually performed on a special tilt table that positions the patient with the head down and butt up-excellent test to examine for an anal fissure or hemorrhoids.

Capsule endoscopy

Procedure in which a tiny camera is ingested to investigate the esophagus and small bowel.

Chronic

Usually refers to a disease that develops slowly and lasts for a long time.

Sigmoidoscopy: performed with or without sedation, this is a "short" colonoscopy used to examine the rectum and left colon.

Proctoscopy: performed without sedation, usually on a special tilt table that positions the patient with the head down and butt up; in this procedure a rigid, straight, lighted tube is used to examine the rectum. While this procedure has mostly been replaced by flexible sigmoidoscopy, this is still an excellent test to examine the rectum.

Anoscopy: performed without sedation, usually on a special tilt table that positions the patient with the head down and butt up. In this procedure a rigid, short, straight, lighted tube is used to examine the anal canal. This is an excellent test to examine for an anal fissure, or hemorrhoids.

Enteroscopy: performed under sedation, a small, thin, long, flexible, lighted tube with a camera on the end is passed through the mouth into the esophagus, stomach, duodenum, and jejunum. This is an excellent test to detect inflammation and strictures in the upper GI tract and upper small intestine.

Capsule endoscopy: performed without sedation, the patient swallows a large pill containing a camera, and wears a sensor device on the abdomen. The capsule passes naturally through the small intestine while transmitting video images to the sensor which stores the data and can be downloaded to a computer for your physician to review. This test is mostly used in evaluating patients with **chronic** gastrointestinal bleeding of obscure origin. Capsule endoscopy is not commonly used in the evaluation of Crohn's disease because other, simpler tests are usually more accurate in diagnosing and assessing the extent and severity of the disease. In addition, the capsule, which is very large, can easily become lodged in an intestinal stricture and cause an obstruction; the patient would need an operation to remove the capsule.

ERCP: performed under sedation, this is an endoscopic procedure used to examine the bile duct and pancreatic duct. This procedure is performed for a variety of reasons including detection and removal of stones in the bile duct, detection of **tumors** involving the bile duct and pancreatic duct, and diagnosis of primary sclerosing **cholangitis**.

3. I am often constipated—should I discuss this with my doctor?

Constipation is defined as having fewer than three bowel movements a week. Other definitions include having hard stools, straining to have a bowel movement, and the sensation of incomplete evacuation. Constipation is a **symptom** and not a disease and most often it is temporary and not serious. It is very common and is usually caused by too little fiber or not enough water in your diet. By better understanding contributing factors, you may be able to change your lifestyle, thereby preventing or minimizing future episodes of constipation.

Most everyone will suffer from constipation at some point in their life. It is estimated that 4 million Americans have constipation and it accounts for 2.5 million physician visits per year. Women are more likely than men to suffer from constipation. It is also a problem more commonly seen in adults, specifically those over the age of 65.

To better understand why constipation occurs, it is helpful to understand the function of the colon or large bowel. By the time material enters the colon from the

Tumor
An abnormal growth of tissue; can be benign or malignant.

Cholangitis
An inflammation of the bile ducts caused by bacteria.

Constipation
Having fewer than three bowel movements per week. It can also be defined as having hard stools or straining to have a bowel movement.

Symptom
Subjective evidence for disease; something that the patient feels.

It is estimated that 4 million Americans have constipation and it accounts for 2.5 million physician visits per year.

small intestine essential nutrients have already been absorbed. The colon functions by removing water from material while it forms waste or stool. Constipation can occur when too much water has been removed or the muscles involved in propelling waste through the colon are slow or abnormal.

Common causes of constipation:

1. Not enough fiber
2. Not enough liquids
3. Limited physical activity
4. Medications like pain medicines, iron supplements, blood pressure medications (calcium channel blockers) and antidepressants
5. Other medical conditions like pregnancy, surgery, **diabetes,** and thyroid disease
6. Problems with the colon-like scar tissue from prior surgery (**adhesions**) and **diverticulosis**
7. Ignoring the urge to defecate can cause loss of this "signal" telling an individual they need to defecate—resulting in constipation
8. A problem with the colon or rectum related to mechanical obstruction can produce constipation. Mechanical obstruction can occur if there is a narrowing or blockage of the colon preventing the normal passage of stool. Conditions that can cause obstruction can include **diverticulitis**, colon **cancer**, and inflammatory bowel disease like Crohn's Disease or scar tissue (adhesive disease).

How is constipation evaluated? A doctor will take a careful history. You may be diagnosed with constipation if you have had at least two of these symptoms for more than twelve weeks within the past twelve months including:

Diabetes

Elevated blood sugar (glucose).

Adhesions

Formation of scar tissue, usually occurring after surgery.

Diverticulosis

Outpouchings in the lining of the colon. When these become inflamed, they can produce symptoms of abdominal pain and fever.

Diverticulitis

An infection of a Diverticulum. This infection can cause a "micro" perforation or tiny hole in the colon wall and create a pocket of pus or abscess.

Cancer

An uncontrollable growth of cells in the body that can spread, or metastasize, to other areas of the body.

1. Straining when moving your bowels

2. Hard or firm stool

3. Feeling of incomplete bowel movements

4. Feeling of blockage in the rectum

5. Less than three bowel movements per week.

Your doctor may perform a digital rectal exam to check for blood. Blood tests to evaluate for **anemia**, thyroid studies, calcium levels and electrolytes may be recommended.

Due to the risk of colon cancer with age, a colonoscopy or barium X-ray of the colon may be performed.

If these tests are normal your doctor may want to do a more detailed testing of the colon to evaluate its function including a **transit study** to make sure the colon is propelling fecal material properly.

Evaluation of the muscles of the **anus** or rectum involved in defecation may be performed with anorectal manometry or balloon expulsion tests. Anorectal manometry evaluates the anal sphincter muscle function and motility of the rectum. In a balloon expulsion test, a balloon is placed in the rectum and slowly inflated. The inflated balloon is meant to simulate stool in the rectum. If you sense rectal fullness with the balloon only minimally inflated, then you have a very sensitive rectum. On the other hand, if the balloon needs to be maximally inflated, then it suggests that your rectum does not sense the presence of stool.

Treatment of constipation depends on the cause. The addition of **fiber** to your diet may be enough to improve symptoms of constipation. It is recommended that you have approximately 30–35 grams of fiber daily to help bulk up and soften your stool. Foods high in fiber

Anemia

A term used to refer to low red blood cell count.

Transit study

A study to evaluate the function of the colon using small capsules that can be see on X-ray.

Anus

The outside opening of the rectum.

Fiber

A substance in foods that comes from plants—helps with digestion by keeping stool soft.

Foods high in fiber include fresh fruits and vegetables and whole grain and bran cereals.

Laxative

Something that loosens the bowels.

include fresh fruits and vegetables and whole grain and bran cereals. Drinking plenty of liquids and avoiding caffeinated beverages, which can be dehydrating, may help relieve constipation.

Laxatives used for a short period of time may be recommended by your doctor to relieve occasional constipation. There are many types of laxatives, which work in different ways.

- *Bulk forming agents* like Metamucil or Citrucel or fiber supplements taken with water absorb extra water in the intestine producing soft bulkier stool.

- *Stimulants* produce contractions of the muscles of the intestines. Medications like Senokot, Correctol, and Dulcolax are stimulants. It is recommended that medications only be used for occasional constipation.

- *Osmotics* cause fluid to be drawn into the colon. These types of medications are used commonly to cleanse the colon in preparation for colonoscopy though they may be used in patients with chronic constipation. Miralax or polyethylene glycol is an example of an osmotic laxative.

- *Stool softeners* work to moisten the stool. An example of a stool softener is Colace. These medications are commonly prescribed after surgery to prevent straining.

- *Chloride channel activators:* These medications work by increasing fluid in your intestine making it easier for the passage of stool. Amitiza or lubiprostone is a chloride channel activator.

- *Lubricating agents* like mineral oil lubricate the stool making it easier to pass through the colon.

4. I often have diarrhea—what does this mean?

Diarrhea is an increase in stool volume or the frequency of bowel movements occurring more than three times a day. Often it is **acute** and self limiting—lasting a few days and resolving spontaneously without any treatment. Chronic diarrhea, defined as ongoing for more than three weeks, may be a sign of a more serious problem. In addition to change in stool volume or frequency, patients with diarrhea may experience abdominal pain, fever, and bleeding with bowel movements.

Acute

Sudden or severe onset.

Common causes of diarrhea include:

- Viral infections like Rotavirus and Norwalk virus commonly referred to as "stomach flu."

- Bacterial infections caused by *Salmonella*, *Shigella*, and *Escherichia coli* (commonly know as E coli) are the result of consuming contaminated food or water.

- Parasites like *Giardia* and *Cryptosporidium* enter the digestive tract through contaminated food or water.

- Medications, including antibiotics, can cause diarrhea. Antibiotic associated diarrhea is the result of an antibiotic altering the bacteria normally present in the intestine. **Clostridium difficile (*C. diff.*)** is a bacterial infection that produces diarrhea that can occur after taking an antibiotic.

- Inflammatory bowel diseases like Crohn's disease or ulcerative **colitis** are inflammatory disorders of the intestinal track that can produce chronic diarrhea. **Celiac disease,** which is an allergy to foods containing gluten, can also be a cause of chronic diarrhea.

Clostridium difficile (*C. diff.*)

Bacterial infection that produces diarrhea that can occur after taking an antibiotic.

Colitis

Inflammation of the colon; can be due to Crohn's disease, ulcerative colitis, or other diseases.

Celiac disease

Hereditary disorder that involves intolerance to gluten, a protein found in wheat, barley, and rye.

11

Chronic pancreatitis

Ongoing inflammation of the pancreas, most often caused by alcohol, although in many cases the cause is unknown.

Malabsorption

A condition in which the small intestine is not able to absorb nutrients and vitamins.

Irritable bowel syndrome

Symptoms of diarrhea in the absense of disease pathology.

- Medical conditions like diabetes or **chronic pancreatitis** can lead to diarrhea as a result of **malabsorption** of nutrients. Individuals with pancreatitis may not produce sufficient enzymes necessary for breakdown and digestion of proteins resulting in diarrhea. Patients with diabetes may have dysmotility of the intestine resulting in proliferation of bacteria to abnormal levels in the intestine resulting in diarrhea.

- **Irritable bowel syndrome** can produce symptoms of diarrhea in the absence of disease pathology. Diarrhea due to irritable bowel syndrome may be strongly influenced by diet, activity, and stress.

Evaluation and Management of Diarrhea

Often acute diarrhea does not warrant evaluation or referral to a physician because symptoms are self-limiting and resolve spontaneously without medical treatment. When symptoms persist, a careful history regarding recent travel, sick contacts, or medication use should be obtained. Collection of the stool can be performed to evaluate for the presence of an infectious etiology. In some cases endoscopic evaluation with sigmoidoscopy or colonoscopy may be necessary to evaluate for inflammatory bowel disease. Treatment is determined by the cause of diarrhea. If an infectious source is suspected and symptoms are not self-limiting, a course of antibiotics may be recommended. There are very effective medications used to treat ulcerative colitis and Crohn's disease if inflammatory bowel disease is the cause of diarrhea. Malabsorption of nutrients causing diarrhea, which can occur in individuals with diabetes or chronic pancreatitis, may be managed with antibiotics or enzyme replacement therapy respectively.

5. *How would I know if I am bleeding from my intestines?*

Acute gastrointestinal bleeding may present as vomiting up blood or material that has a "coffee grounds" appearance. Bloody bowel movements or black or tarry stool may also be present. Associated symptoms may include abdominal pain, weakness, or lightheadedness. Individuals with heart disease may also experience chest pain or shortness of breath.

Vomiting of blood usually originates from an upper gastrointestinal source, whereas bright red blood or maroon stool can be from either a lower gastrointestinal source, such as the rectum or colon, or from brisk bleeding from an upper gastrointestinal source.

Long-term gastrointestinal bleeding may go unnoticed because small amounts of blood are lost via the gastrointestinal tract and may not be visible to the eye. This is called occult blood loss. Symptoms may include pale skin color, fatigue, and shortness of breath. Long-term gastrointestinal bleeding can be diagnosed by a blood test or an examination of the stool for trace amounts of blood.

Causes of upper gastrointestinal bleeding include:

- Peptic **ulcer** disease
- Gastritis or inflammation of the lining of the stomach
- Esophageal or gastric **varices**—a condition seen in patients with chronic liver disease.
- Mallory-Weiss Tears—small tear or laceration of the lining of the esophagus or stomach associated with retching

Ulcer

An area of damage or a break in the lining of the gut.

Varices

Abnormal blood vessels that can form in the esophagus and stomach in a patient with liver disease that can lead to gastrointestinal bleeding.

Causes of lower gastrointestinal bleeding include:

- Diverticulosis, small outpouchings in the lining of the colon wall, are the most common cause of lower gastrointestinal bleeding. Bleeding is usually painless and bright red or maroon in color.
- Angiodysplasia,abnormal or malformed blood vessels, can form anywhere in the gastrointestinal tract with the colon being the most common site. They are more commonly seen in older patients and in patients with chronic kidney disease.
- **Polyps**, colon cancer, and noncancerous growth in the colon that can lead to colon cancer, can cause both acute and chronic gastrointestinal bleeding.
- **Hemorrhoids** and anal fissures—Hemorrhoids are engorgement of veins in the rectum that can occur as a result of straining with bowel movements and constipation. **Fissure** is a tear in the lining of the anal wall usually due to straining during bowel movements which associated pain and bleeding.

When should you seek medical attention? Any gastrointestinal bleeding requires immediate medical attention. Individuals experiencing any of the symptoms should consult with their doctor.

6. I have been unintentionally losing weight—should I tell my doctor?

Unintentional weight loss or loss of weight that is not the result of diet or exercise may be a sign of an underlying medical condition. Possible gastrointestinal causes of unintentional weight loss can include:

- Inability to chew—may be caused by poor dentition, mouth sores, or non-fitting dentures.

Polyps

Growths of the lining of the colon that are benign or premalignant.

Hemorrhoids

Inflammation of the blood vessels around the anus or lower rectum.

Fissure

A crack or split most often seen in the anal canal.

Any gastro-intestinal bleeding requires immediate medical attention.

- Difficulty swallowing—disorder of the esophagus which produces difficulty swallowing is called **dysphagia**. This can be due to a narrowing of the esophagus, such as a stricture, or certain diseases, such as **achalasia** or **scleroderma**.

- Peptic ulcer disease—including stomach or duodenal ulcers, or even chronic gastritis, may produce early satiety, which is the sensation that one fills up quickly with only small amounts of food.

- Anorexia—loss of appetite that may be caused by depression, eating disorders including anorexia nervosa and bulimia, acute and chronic infections, pregnancy, cancer, thyroid disease or medications.

- Diarrhea—This is a symptom of a disease, rather than a disease itself. Some causes of diarrhea include viral, bacterial, or parasitic infections, and inflammatory bowel diseases including Crohn's disease and ulcerative colitis.

- Malabsorptive syndromes—inability to digest food or certain types of food results in damage to the lining of the small intestine preventing absorption of nutrients. Celiac disease is an example of a malabsorptive syndrome.

- Hormone secreting tumors—Zollinger-Ellison Syndrome is caused by abnormal production of the hormone gastrin which is produced by a small tumor usually in the pancreas or small bowel or intestine. Carcinoid tumors are tumors which can occur in the small intestine, colon, airways or appendix. Carcinoid tumors produce excessive amounts of the hormone serotonin, which can cause flushing, diarrhea, and weight loss.

Dysphagia

Difficulty swallowing; the sensation during swallowing of food getting stuck somewhere in the neck or chest.

Achalasia

A motility disorder of the esophagus producing symptoms of difficulty swallowing.

Scleroderma

An autoimmune condition that can affect any part of the body and is characterized by thickening and scarring of affected organs.

15

7. I have bloating and gas—what does this mean, and should I be concerned?

Gas is normal. Everyone has it and eliminates it by burping or passing it through the rectum. On average, an individual will produce several pints of gas a day and pass gas about a dozen times a day. Though gas formation and passage is common, it can be uncomfortable and embarrassing. By understanding what contributes to gas formation you can make changes in life style and eating habits to help improve symptoms.

Gas is mostly odorless and composed of oxygen, nitrogen, carbon dioxide, and methane. Gas comes from two sources: either swallowed air or a by-product of digested food. The unpleasant odor experienced with flatulence is caused by bacteria. Bacteria breakdown food and produce sulfur-containing gas which then is expelled.

Swallowing air is a frequent cause of gas in the stomach. Small amounts of air are swallowed when you drink and eat, especially if you eat quickly. Most of the air that is swallowed is released by burping. Gas that remains passes into the bowel where some of it is absorbed. The gas that is not absorbed will be passed out though the rectum.

Undigested food that is not absorbed by the small intestine passes into the colon or large bowel. In the colon, the normal presence of bacteria will work to break down any remaining material, which produces hydrogen, carbon dioxide, and sometimes methane.

Foods containing sugar or carbohydrates produce excess amounts of gas, while foods containing a higher percentage of fats and proteins cause little gas production. In addition, foods that are not well digested—like broccoli or cabbage as well as high fiber foods like bran and oats—can contribute to gas production. Lactose is a sugar found in milk products like ice cream and cheese. When lactase, the enzyme necessary to digest milk products, is absent or produced in diminished levels, undigested sugars pass into the colon causing gas and bloating. If your doctor suspects lactase deficiency as a cause of your gas, a breath test can be performed to find out if you are lactose intolerant. The breath test detects excess amounts of hydrogen released by bacteria as the undigested lactose ferments in the colon or large bowel.

Excess gas or belching may be caused by gastritis or inflammation of the lining of the stomach. Infection with the bacteria *Helicobacter pylori* is a common cause of gastritis. Presence of *Helicobacter pylori* can be determined by endoscopy, blood test, or breath test. If *Helicobacter pylori* is present and contributing to your symptoms, your doctor may prescribe a treatment plan that includes a combination of antibiotics and acid blocking medication.

Helicobacter pylori (H. pylori)

A bacterium that lives in the stomach and can cause stomach ulcers.

Treatment of excessive bloating and gas often includes altering your diet, reducing the amount of air swallowed, and sometimes taking medication. Avoiding foods which are gas producing may reduce symptoms.

For individuals with **lactose intolerance**, replacement with the over-the-counter enzyme lactase will aid in lactose digestion. Lactase enzyme replacement is available in a caplet or chewable tablet that can be taken before eating lactose-containing foods. Reduced or lactose free milk and dairy products are also readily available.

Lactose intolerance

Common disorder caused by lack of a digestive enzyme that normally breaks down sugars found in milk resulting in diarrhea, cramps, and gas.

8. What is irritable bowel syndrome and how is it treated?

Irritable bowel syndrome, or IBS, is a common disorder of the intestine, producing symptoms of abdominal pain, excessive gas, diarrhea, or constipation. IBS can be a cause of chronic abdominal pain but does not harm the intestines or lead to serious disease. Things like stress, activity level, and diet can produce symptoms. Most individuals can control their symptoms with diet, stress reduction, and medications prescribed by your doctor. For some people, IBS can be very debilitating and have considerable effect on an individual's quality of life.

It is estimated that 20% of adults suffer from symptoms related to IBS on a regular basis.

IBS is very common. It is estimated that 20% of adults suffer from symptoms related to IBS on a regular basis. It occurs more commonly in women than men and typically occurs before the age of 35, although it can be seen at any age.

Symptoms most commonly associated with IBS include abdominal pain, bloating, and discomfort. Some individuals may have constipation, which involves hard and difficult to pass bowel movements. If you are constipated, you may have straining and cramping when trying to have a bowel movement. Sometimes mucus will be seen in the bowel movements, which is a fluid that helps to moisten the bowel movements as they move through the intestinal tract. Conversely, some people with IBS may have diarrhea, which is loose, watery stools. People with diarrhea may have **urgency**—the sensation that they may have a bowel movement that they cannot control. Individuals with IBS may also alternate between constipation and diarrhea.

Urgency
The feeling that one has to move their bowels or urinate right away.

Doctors have not discovered a specific cause for IBS. Some medical experts believe that individuals with IBS have an intestine that is overly sensitive and reactive to certain foods and stress. Others believe that IBS may sometimes develop after someone has had an infection in the bowel; this is called post-infectious IBS.

Serotonin, which is a chemical that transmits information from one part of the body to another, can be found in the brain and gastrointestinal tract. If you have IBS, you may have increased levels of serotonin, which means you have more sensitive pain sensors in the gastrointestinal tract and therefore experience problems with bowel movements and sensation.

Some people with IBS also suffer from depression and anxiety, making the symptoms worse. Also, the symptoms of IBS can cause a person to feel anxious or depressed.

Some medical conditions have been described with increased frequency in patients with IBS. As example, scientists have found celiac disease in people with similar symptoms to IBS. People with celiac disease have an allergy to gluten, which is a protein found in wheat, rye, and barley. Individuals with celiac disease become sick if they ingest gluten-containing foods. A reliable blood test is available to check for celiac disease.

There is no particular test to diagnose IBS. Your doctor will take a careful history and may schedule you for blood tests, stool samples, and X-rays. Often a doctor will perform a sigmoidoscopy or colonoscopy. If your tests are negative your doctor may diagnose you with IBS.

There is no cure for IBS. Changes in behavior may improve the symptoms, including reduction in stress and change in diet. Medications are an important part of relieving symptoms. Your doctor may recommend a fiber supplement or laxative for constipation or a medication to relieve diarrhea. Other medications may include antispasmodics to relieve spasm in the colon associated with abdominal pain. Medications that relax the bowel may also be used to relieve symptoms. There are medications specifically used to treat IBS. If your symptoms are primarily constipation or diarrhea your doctor may suggest a trial of a medication.

9. I think that my skin is yellow— what does this mean?

Jaundice

Yellowing of the skin due to buildup of bile. The most common causes of jaundice are hepatitis (infection of the liver), and blockage of the outflow of bile from the liver into the intestine from either a stone in the bile duct or a tumor.

Bilirubin

Product of the breakdown of hemoglobin, which can be measured to evaluate the liver and gall bladder.

Cells

The smallest unit in the body; millions of cells attached together make up our organs and tissues.

Jaundice, or yellowing of the skin, is not a disease but a sign that can occur in different diseases. Jaundice occurs when **bilirubin** accumulates under the skin turning it yellow or brown.

Bilirubin comes from red blood **cells**. Red blood cells become fragile as they get older and are destroyed by the body. Bilirubin that is released from red blood cells is removed from blood by the liver.

The liver has many functions. One function of the liver is to produce and release bile into the small intestine that helps in fat digestion. The liver also plays an important role in clearing the body of toxins and waste that the body produces—like bilirubin.

Jaundice can occur when there is:

- Too much bilirubin being produced from the blood for the liver to remove (increased red blood cell destruction)
- A problem with the liver's ability to remove and process the bilirubin (inflammation of the liver)

- A problem with blockage of the bile ducts which forces bilirubin to exit the liver and pass into the small intestine. This can occur with gallstones that have migrated from the gallbladder into the bile duct, or from inflammation of the bile ducts.

In addition to turning the skin yellow, jaundice can cause the stool to become light or "clay colored." This occurs due to the absence of bilirubin in the stool, which normally turns it a brown color. The urine may also turn dark. This happens when the bilirubin starts to accumulate in the blood and is excreted by the kidney turning the urine brown.

If jaundice is due to a liver problem, a person may experience fatigue, poor appetite, swelling of the abdomen and ankles, confusion, and sometimes bleeding from the intestines.

If jaundice is due to the blockage of bile ducts and fat digestion is impaired; the body cannot absorb some vitamins and nutrients. Vitamin K in particular is dependent on the presence of bilirubin for its absorption. Vitamin K plays an important role in blood clotting. In the absence of vitamin K, individuals can have a tendency to bleed excessively from a small cut.

Many diseases can cause jaundice. Any condition in which the liver becomes inflamed (**hepatitis**) may affect the liver's ability to function resulting in yellowing of the skin. Common examples include viruses, alcohol, or acetaminophen (Tylenol).

Chronic conditions of the liver can lead to long-term damage of the liver (**cirrhosis**) resulting in jaundice. Common examples include hepatitis C, alcohol related

Hepatitis

Inflammation of the liver that causes cell damage.

Cirrhosis

Formation of permanent scar tissue in the liver due to a chronic condition.

21

Autoimmune hepatitis

A liver disease characterized by an overactive immune system that attacks the liver.

The cause of jaundice is best evaluated by a careful history and examination.

Liver biopsy

A test where a small needle is passed into the liver and a piece of the liver is removed and examined under a microscope.

Dehydration

Reduction of water content.

Hyperemesis gravidarum

Severe nausea and vomiting typically occurring during the beginning stages of pregnancy.

cirrhosis, iron overload (hemochromatosis), and **autoimmune hepatitis**.

Medications may cause inflammation of the liver, resulting in jaundice. Most often the treatment is discontinuation of the medication. In some cases, it may take several weeks to months before the jaundice resolves.

The cause of jaundice is best evaluated by a careful history and examination. Regular heavy alcohol use may point to alcohol related injury. Use of illicit injectable drugs may suggest viral hepatitis. New medication use may point to drug induced hepatitis.

Simple blood tests and abdominal imaging like an ultrasound, computerized tomography, or magnetic resonance imaging may be performed.

In some cases a **liver biopsy** may be suggested if the cause of the jaundice cannot be determined. A liver biopsy is performed using a local anesthetic to numb the skin and then inserting a needle into the liver, allowing the physician to remove a small piece of tissue that will then be looked at under a microscope.

10. I am pregnant—can this affect my digestive health?

Morning sickness, or mild nausea or vomiting caused by pregnancy, typically occurs during the first trimester in about 50–90% of all pregnancies. Thought it is commonly seen in the beginning stages of pregnancy, symptoms can continue into the third trimester. When it is severe—associated with weight loss and **dehydration**— it is referred to as **hyperemesis gravidarum**. Morning sickness is a misnomer; as symptoms can occur at any time and persist throughout the day.

The cause of morning sickness is unknown. It is thought that hormonal changes occurring during pregnancy may play a role. Abnormal stomach emptying or gastric motility may also contribute to nausea and vomiting during pregnancy.

Treatment is supportive and symptoms usually resolve by the second trimester. Simply limiting oral intake during episodes and reintroducing liquids when symptoms have passed is sufficient. When it is severe, resuscitation with intravenous fluids may be necessary.

Pregnancy can have many different effects on the gastrointestinal tract. **Heartburn** or gastroesophageal **reflux** disease is the most common GI complaint seen during pregnancy and can occur in upwards of 50% of pregnant woman. Lifestyle modifications like elevating the head of the bed, eating small frequent meals, and refraining from eating at least three hours before bedtime may improve heartburn symptoms. While lifestyle modifications may help improve symptoms, most patients require treatment with an acid blocking medication. There are medications that are safe to take during pregnancy that your doctor may prescribe.

Heartburn

The sensation of burning discomfort or warmth traveling up from the stomach into the chest. A symptom of GERD.

Reflux

The movement of food, fluid, or acid up from the stomach into the esophagus.

Gas, bloating, and constipation commonly occur during pregnancy. Pregnancy hormones may affect motility of the intestine, contributing to these symptoms. To manage constipation, your doctor may suggest increasing your fiber intake or taking a fiber supplement.

Hemorrhoids are engorged blood vessels in the rectum caused by increased pressure. Hemorrhoids can occur throughout pregnancy but are most common in the third trimester and occur in upwards of 30–40% of pregnant women. Hemorrhoids can occur during pregnancy due to pressure an enlarged uterus places on the large vein (inferior vena cava) that is responsible for drainage of veins of the colon and rectum. Hemorrhoids can produce bleeding, pain, and itching. Hemorrhoids occurring during pregnancy usually get better after giving birth.

Constipation can make hemorrhoids worse. Iron, which is found in prenatal vitamins, causes constipation and can make symptoms of hard or infrequent bowel movements worse.

Treatment of constipation and hemorrhoids includes a diet high in fiber and drinking plenty of liquids. A stool softener may also prevent straining.

Keeping the anus clean after each bowel movement can treat itching or pain related to hemorrhoids. Taking a warm soak in a tub may relieve discomfort and help shrink the hemorrhoids. Treatment may also consist of a local anti-inflammatory preparation placed on the hemorrhoid.

Intrahepatic cholestasis of pregnancy

Itching and yellowing of the skin usually occurring during the late stages of pregnancy.

HELLP syndrome (Hemolysis, Elevated Liver Enzymes, and Low Platelets)

Life threatening condition occurring during the later stages of pregnancy.

In rare situations, the liver may become inflamed during pregnancy. Liver diseases that are specific to pregnancy include **intrahepatic cholestasis of pregnancy** and **acute fatty liver of pregnancy**. **HELLP** syndrome or Hemolysis, Elevated Liver enzymes and Low Platelets is also a disease unique to pregnancy that can affect the liver. Hepatitis associated with pregnancy may produce symptoms of yellow skin, itching, abdominal pain, nausea, and vomiting. These are potentially serious conditions that should be carefully evaluated by a physician.

11. Can medications affect my digestive system?

Medications taken by mouth are generally very safe and well tolerated by most people. Both prescription and over-the-counter drugs may have adverse or undesirable effects in some individuals. Generally these **side effects** are mild and tolerable but in rare situations may cause significant toxicity and pose potential harm to an individual. You should inform you physician of any possible drug allergies or history of intolerance to certain medications.

Medication-Induced Esophageal Injury

Some people have a difficult time swallowing medications. Pills or capsules that remain in the esophagus can cause injury and produce painful swallowing. Chronic medical conditions like scleroderma and achalasia, which can affect the motility or passage of food in the esophagus, may increase the risk of medication induced esophageal injuries. These injuries can include the development of ulcers, bleeding, and in rare cases, perforation. Medications commonly associated with injuries to the esophagus are aspirin, potassium supplements, antibiotics, and medications for **osteoporosis**.

Some medications may affect the muscle or sphincter between the esophagus and stomach. This muscle normally relaxes when we eat and swallow. Some medications may increase relaxation of this muscle producing heartburn or reflux symptoms. Medications that may cause reflux include blood pressure medications, like nitrates and calcium channel blockers, and asthma medications like theophylline and anticholinergic medications.

Side effect

An adverse reaction to a medication or treatment.

Osteoporosis

A severe decrease in bone density; can be seen after long-term use of corticosteroids.

Some medications may affect the muscle or sphincter between the esophagus and stomach.

There are a number of lifestyle changes a person can do to reduce the chance on medication induced esophageal injury:

1. Take all medications with plenty of liquids.
2. Make sure you are able to sit or stand before taking certain medications.
3. Do not lie down for a minimum of 30 minutes after taking certain medications.

Medication-Induced Stomach Injury

Medications like aspirin and nonsteroidal anti-inflammatory medication (NSAIDS) including ibuprofen and naprosyn can produce ulcers in the lining of the stomach and small intestine. These medications can cause pain, bleeding, and in some cases perforation of the lining of the intestine. To minimize the risk of developing an ulcer you can:

1. Take coated or enteric aspirin, which may reduce the risk of stomach irritation.
2. Avoid alcoholic beverages when taking these medications.
3. Avoid taking these medications on a regular basis unless instructed by a physician.
4. Take an **antacid** when taking these medications to reduce the risk of stomach irritation.

Medication-Induced Constipation

Many medications affect the motility of the colon. Medication induced constipation is very common, resulting in slow transit or passage of stool in the colon. Medications commonly producing constipation include iron or iron containing vitamins, blood pressure medication, pain medications, and cholesterol lowering drugs. To minimize constipation due to medications you should:

Antacid

A medication available over the counter, effective for active symptoms of reflux. Antacids work by neutralizing acid on contact. Many types are available without a doctor's prescription.

1. Drink plenty of liquids.

2. Eat a diet high in fiber, including whole grains, fruits, and vegetables.

3. Get plenty of exercise.

Medication-Induced Diarrhea

Antibiotics are the most common medications associated with diarrhea. Antibiotics can alter the bacteria normally present in the gastrointestinal tract resulting in **bacterial overgrowth**. Antibiotics like clindamycin, ampicillin, and cephalosporins are the most common medications to cause diarrhea.

Bacterial overgrowth

A condition in which there is an overgrowth of normal intestinal flora; usually seen in the setting of an intestinal stricture.

27

PART TWO

The Esophagus, Stomach, and Acid-Related Disorders

Stephen F. Nezhad, MD

What is an ulcer?

How do you treat *H. pylori*?

I have frequent heartburn—
does this mean I have GERD
(Gastroesophageal reflux disease)?

More . . .

12. What is an ulcer?

An ulcer is a crater that can form in the lining of the stomach or the intestine. The lining of the stomach and intestine is called the mucosa. Breaks in the lining of the mucosa can occur for a variety of reasons. Breaks that are smaller than five mm are called erosions. Breaks larger than five mm are called ulcers. Ulcers can vary in size from the size of a nickel to larger than a half dollar. They can occur anywhere in the gastrointestinal tract from the mouth to the anus. Most occur in the stomach or in the first six inches of the small intestine, called the duodenum.

There are many causes of ulcers. The two most common causes of ulcers include anti-inflammatory medications and an infection with a bacterium called *Helicobacter pylori*, or *H. pylori*. Anti-inflammatory medications include aspirin, ibuprofen, and naproxen. The excessive use of these medications can cause an ulcer. Acetaminophen, or Tylenol, , on the other hand, does not cause ulcers. *H. pylori* is a bacterium, or germ, that can also cause ulcers in the stomach and duodenum. This bacterium can survive the acidic environment of the stomach and cause a breakdown in the production of protective mucus, leading to ulcers. Stress does not cause ulcers but can delay healing. Similarly, smoking tobacco and excess alcohol can delay healing of stomach ulcers. Most ulcers are not cancerous, but certain ones in the stomach can become cancerous and need to be followed by your doctor.

More than 4 million people suffer from stomach ulcers each year.

Ulcers are very common in the United States. More than 4 million people suffer from stomach ulcers each year. An estimated 5.65 billion dollars are spent annually in this country alone on ulcers. This includes money spent on hospitalization, treatment, and potential lost revenue from work. This figure does not include the costs for medications to treat ulcers, which are significant as well.

13. How do I know if I have an ulcer?

Ulcers can cause a variety of symptoms depending on their size. Small ulcers can be painless and can have no symptoms whatsoever. Large ulcers can cause pain or bleeding. The pain from an ulcer is typically a gnawing or burning ache in the upper abdomen. It can last from 30 minutes to over two hours. It can even awaken people from sleeping. Patients may complain of a "raw" stomach or have hunger pains. It is common for people with ulcers to experience this type of pain two to five hours after eating. Another common time to experience this pain is at night. The stomach produces the largest amount of acid between 11 PM and 2 AM. Symptoms commonly occur during this time in people with ulcers. Other, less common ulcer symptoms include nausea, loss of appetite, and even weight loss.

Eating food or drinking milk can ease the pain from an ulcer. Before antacids, many patients were told by their doctors to follow the Sippy diet to heal an ulcer. This is a diet designed to neutralize the acidity of gastric juice. It consists of a combination of milk, cream, and bland foods. Alkaline powders were also used in combination with this diet. This diet is no longer used since there are powerful medications that can cure ulcers.

If an ulcer grows large, it can rupture an adjacent blood vessel and cause bleeding. Bleeding in the stomach can cause nausea and vomiting of blood. As blood goes down the gastrointestinal tract it is digested and turns color from red to black. Black stools can sometimes be the only sign of a bleeding ulcer. This is a very serious sign. Your doctor needs to know if this happens and would want to check you for internal bleeding.

Large ulcers can cause swelling of the adjacent tissues resulting in obstruction, or a blockage of the intestine. This can prevent food from passing through the digestive tract resulting in vomiting and weight loss. As an ulcer heals it can also create a blockage by forming scar tissue around it, which narrows the digestive tract, resulting in similar symptoms. This can require surgery to remove the scarred segment of bowel.

Rarely, an ulcer can go all the way through the stomach and cause a hole, or perforation, leading to a rupture of the bowel and **peritonitis**. This causes severe pain and fever. Almost all perforated ulcers need an operation to fix and can sometimes cause death. About 6000 people die each year in the United States from the complications of an ulcer.

Peritonitis

Inflammation of the lining that surrounds organs in the abdominal cavity.

14. How do you test for an ulcer?

Tests for an ulcer include an X-ray of the stomach, called an upper gastrointestinal series (upper GI series), or an exam with a camera, or **endoscope**, called an upper endoscopy. The upper GI series involves a patient drinking a thick white shake of barium. This coats the stomach and identifies ulcers by X-ray. It is painless. The barium will eventually pass in your stool. The advantage of an upper GI series is that it is a non-invasive test and extremely safe. A patient can drive after the test.

Endoscope

Thin, flexible tube with an attached light that is used to view the digestive tract.

An endoscopy involves having an endoscope passed into the mouth, through the esophagus, and into the stomach. The endoscope is a long slender tube, the thickness of an adult's pinky finger. At the tip of the tube is a light and a video chip which transmits the images to a monitor where your doctor can watch and steer the camera so that the entire stomach is seen. Patients are sedated for this exam, which is painless and takes about 20 minutes to perform. Afterwards, some patients may experience a sore throat for a few hours but most feel nothing at all. Patients receive relaxing medications prior to an upper endoscopy to make them comfortable for the exam. However, patients cannot drive afterwards. An advantage of an endoscopy is that it allows your doctor to obtain tissue samples, or biopsies, of the stomach. This can check for infection with *H. pylori* and to see if the ulcer is cancerous.

Bleeding ulcers are treated very seriously. This is a common reason for people to be admitted to hospitals. If there has been significant blood loss, a patient may have a rapid heart rate and low blood pressure. In the emergency room, patients are given intravenous fluid to raise the blood pressure. Blood counts are checked and if low, a blood transfusion may be necessary.

Sometimes an upper endoscopy is needed to stop the bleeding. Doctors can pass small instruments through long channels within the scope to deliver a variety of treatments directly to an ulcer. This procedure may save a patient from needing surgery. All of the procedures are very safe and have prevented thousands of patients each year from needing emergency surgery for bleeding ulcers.

15. How do you treat an ulcer?

Nowadays, both over-the-counter and prescription medications are used regularly to relieve the pain from ulcers, indigestion, and gastroesophageal reflux. The two general types of medications commonly used are topical antacids and acid reducing pills. The topical antacids are thick, chalky drinks designed to coat the stomach and soothe the irritation from the ulcer. Aluminum and magnesium hydroxide (Maalox) is a common example. These topical agents usually work the fastest by coating the stomach and buffering the sensitive areas from stomach acid. They generally relieve the symptoms of an ulcer but stronger medicines are needed to actually heal the ulcer. Those stronger medicines are called acid reducing medicines. There are two types of acid reducing medicines: histamine blocking drugs, such as Zantac or Pepcid, and the **proton pump inhibitors**, such as Prilosec or Nexium. Both of these medicines decrease the production of stomach acid and allow ulcers to heal. They are very safe medicines with few side effects. Many are now available over-the-counter. The length of treatment depends on the type of ulcer and is often individualized to the patient. In general, duodenal ulcers are treated for four to six weeks and stomach ulcers for eight weeks. When *H. pylori* is found, antibiotics are needed to both cure the infection and to prevent the ulcer from recurring. This will be discussed in detail in **Questions 16** and **17**.

No specific dietary restrictions are necessary when you have an ulcer but certain foods may worsen ulcer symptoms and should be avoided. These include spicy foods, citrus, and alcohol. Smoking may delay healing of ulcers and is linked to ulcer **recurrence**. Therefore, patients who smoke should stop when an ulcer is diagnosed. It is also important to stop taking anti-inflammatory

Proton pump inhibitor (PPI):

A drug that blocks acid production by the stomach; believed to be stronger and more effective than H2 blockers are.

Recurrence

The reappearance of a disease.

medications as these medications delay ulcer healing. Surgery is rarely needed and is reserved for when ulcers don't heal or if there are complications form ulcers such as bleeding, perforation, or obstruction.

16. *What is* Helicobacter pylori (H. pylori) *and how do I know if I have it?*

H. pylori is a bacterium that lives in the stomach and is one of the most common infections in humans. This bacterium is present in approximately one-half of the world's population. *H. pylori* is common in older adults in this country and less common in children. In the United States, estimates suggest that approximately 40–50% of people have *H. pylori*. *H. pylori* is even more common in adults in underdeveloped countries where up to 75% of people can be infected. The spread or transmission of *H. pylori* is thought to be due to contaminated water supplies and inadequate water treatment facilities.

Most people with *H. pylori* infection have no symptoms. The bacterium can live in the stomach for many years without causing ulcers or any symptoms whatsoever. However, *H. pylori* can cause ulcers of the stomach and duodenum. It lives in the lining of the stomach and can release toxins that damage the mucus-producing cells. This mucus is needed to serve as the protective barrier between the stomach acid and the lining of the stomach. Without it, stomach acid can irritate the lining of the stomach and damage to the lining of the stomach and form an ulcer. This ongoing damage to the stomach lining can increase the risk of developing stomach cancer as well. There is a strong association between *H. pylori* and stomach cancer. Why some people are at

H. pylori *is a bacterium that lives in the stomach and is one of the most common infections in humans.*

risk of these complications from infection with *H. pylori* and others are not is poorly understood and is an area of an intense medical research at the present time.

Antibody

A protein produced the the body's immune system to fight disease.

There are several ways to test for *H. Pylori*. There is a blood test called an **antibody** test. Antibodies are proteins that your body makes when exposed to a foreign substance, such as an infection. If the antibody is present in the blood then you have had or currently have infection with *H. Pylori*. The problem with the antibody test is that it remains positive even after effective treatment for *H. Pylori*.

There is a breath test for *H. Pylori*, which has the advantage of telling you and your doctor if there is an active infection in the stomach. Patients are given a special drink containing a food for the bacterium, called urea. If the bacterium is present in the stomach, the urea is digested by the bacterium and exhaled by the lungs. This can be measured by collecting your breath in a bag and analyzing it for a special gas.

Finally, biopsies of the stomach can be taken to check for *H. Pylori*. This requires an endoscopy by your doctor to look down into the stomach and collect samples to run tests checking for the bacterium. These tests usually require a day or two before the results are known.

17. How do you treat H. pylori?

Risk factor

Things that predispose someone for getting a disease; as example, smoking is a risk factor for lung cancer.

If you have *H. Pylori*, you should be treated. *H. pylori* can cause ulcers and is a **risk factor** for stomach cancer. Infections with *H. pylori* are treated with a two week course of antibiotics. The bacterium is tricky and needs two different antibiotics and an acid-reducing drug, such as Prilosec, in combination to cure it. These medicines are generally pre-packaged for convenience. The combination therapies cost $200 to $300 and are covered by most drug prescription insurance plans. In general, no further testing is necessary after appropriate treatment, since the medicines cure the infection in almost all cases.

18. I have frequent heartburn— does this mean I have GERD (Gastroesophageal reflux disease)?

Classic heartburn is a feeling of burning below the breastbone that comes on after eating or when lying down too soon after eating. It occurs when stomach acid flows back into the esophagus causing irritation and sometimes damage to the lining of the esophagus. Heartburn is extremely common in the United States and it is estimated that over 10 million people feel heartburn every day. The feeling can travel upwards towards your neck and can be associated with a bitter or sour taste in the back of your throat. Other symptoms can include throat clearing, hoarseness, and cough as the acid may irritate the throat and the vocal cords. Heartburn becomes **GERD** when symptoms occur very regularly or when damage occurs in the lining of the esophagus. People who have very bad heartburn, more than three to four times a week, or who have severe heartburn at night, typically have GERD.

GERD
Gastroesophageal reflux disease. A disease made up of symptoms of heartburn, reflux, and/or regurgitation.

19. How do you treat GERD?

There are many ways to treat GERD. First, there are dietary modifications. Many foods can worsen GERD

Lower esophageal sphincter (LES)

A circular muscle at the bottom of the esophagus above the stomach. This muscle opens when food enters the esophagus, allowing the food passage into the stomach, and contracts, or closes, in between swallows. This muscle, or sphincter, may be too loose or may open ay inappropriate times, allowing material to reflux from the stomach up into the esophagus.

by weakening the valve at the bottom of the esophagus called the **lower esophageal sphincter**. This is a round muscle the shape of a doughnut that opens to allow food to pass into the stomach after you swallow. This muscle should stay closed when food is in the stomach so that food and acid do not wash back up into the esophagus. Some foods weaken this muscle. Common dietary triggers for GERD include caffeine, alcohol, chocolate, peppermint, spicy, and fatty foods. Citrus and tomato-based foods may worsen symptoms of GERD as well.

There are many important lifestyle modifications that can minimize GERD symptoms. Stopping smoking can minimize GERD symptoms. Smoking decreases saliva production in the mouth. Saliva is needed to help neutralize stomach acid when it enters the esophagus. Without adequate amounts of saliva, smokers are more likely to suffer from GERD than non-smokers. In addition, smoking weakens the LES making acid reflux more likely in smokers.

Over-eating is another important trigger for GERD. When the stomach is overly distended with food, reflux is more likely to occur. This is especially true in people with a hiatal hernia. The stomach is normally below the diaphragm in the abdomen, and the esophagus is normally above the diaphragm in the chest. The esophagus goes through an opening in the diaphragm where it connects to the stomach. There is a sphincter, or valve, between the esophagus and the stomach called the lower esophageal sphincter. A **hiatal hernia** develops when the opening in the diaphragm where the esophagus meets the stomach becomes larger, and as a result the top of the stomach pushes through the opening into the chest. This causes the valve to become "leaky" and allows stomach acid to reflux into the esophagus more

Hiatal hernia or hiatus hernia

This is the condition where a small or large portion of the stomach, which is usually in the abdomen, pushes through a hole in the diaphragm into the chest. This is often associated with heartburn and GERD.

easily. Eating smaller meals can minimize GERD by putting less pressure on the valve. Hiatal hernias are very common in people over the age of 50. They form when the tissues that hold the stomach in place loosen with age. Unfortunately, there is no way to prevent them from occurring.

People who are overweight tend to have more GERD, so losing weight can help. Other lifestyle modifications include avoiding tight fitting clothes and not eating within two hours of lying down or going to bed. Finally, patients who have GERD during the night may benefit from raising the head of the bed 6 inches to allow gravity to help keep the acid in the stomach and away from the esophagus.

Many patients have persistent symptoms despite dietary and lifestyle modifications. For these patients, medications are usually necessary. In general, there are two types of treatments—topical antacids and acid-reducing medicines. Topical antacids, such as Maalox or Mylanta, work by coating the esophagus with a protective barrier to prevent acid injury. This type of medication works quickly to ease the discomfort of GERD.

Acid-reducing medicines can be divided into two groups, the histamine blockers and the proton pump inhibitors. These medicines typically take longer to work than the topical medications but can provide extended relief of symptoms. Histamine blockers include: ranitidine (Zantac), famotidine (Pepcid), and cimetidine (Tagamet). These medications are usually sufficient for patients with mild to moderate symptoms of GERD. The proton pump inhibitors are the strongest antacids available and work by shutting down the "acid pumps" in the stomach. Without stomach acid there

can be no GERD. These medicines include omeprazole (Prilosec), esomeprazole (Nexium), pantoprazole
(Protonix), lansoprazole (Prevacid), and rabeprazole
(Aciphex). These medicines are very effective in controlling GERD in patients with severe symptoms. Both
the histamine blockers and the proton pump inhibitors
are safe. Many patients have taken these medications for
extended periods of time without side effects.

Occasionally, surgery is recommended for patients with
GERD. Surgery is usually reserved for patients who
have symptoms controlled with medications but prefer
not to take the medications on a long-term basis. The
typical surgery is called a Nissen Fundoplication and
involves the surgeon wrapping the top of the stomach
around the lower esophagus to help close the valve at
the bottom of the esophagus and prevent the stomach
acid from refluxing into the esophagus

**Barrett's
esophagus**

An inflammatory
condition of the
esophagus caused by
chronic gastroesoph-
ageal reflux disease.
Barrett's esophagus
is a more acid-resis-
tant lining of the
esophagus that can
predispose a person
to the development
of esophageal cancer.

Pathologist

A physician trained
in the evaluation of
organs, tissues, and
cells, usually under
a microscope; assists
in determining and
characterizing the
presence of disease.

20. What is Barrett's esophagus?

Barrett's esophagus occurs when the lining at the
bottom of the esophagus is damaged as a result of severe
GERD. It is a rare complication of severe, long-standing GERD. It is painless and does not cause bleeding. It
can occur in men and women who have had many years
of daily, severe, heartburn. The only way your doctor can
tell if you have Barrett's esophagus is by performing an
endoscopy to check you for it. The endoscopy involves
placing a flexible camera into the esophagus and examining the lining of the esophagus for characteristic color
changes. If present, tissue samples, called biopsies, can
be taken to check for changes in the types of cell that
line the esophagus. A **pathologist** can study the samples
under a microscope. Barrett's esophagus occurs when

cells that typically are found lower down in the digestive tract, called intestinal cells, are found in the esophagus and replace the cells that normally reside there, called squamous cells. Doctors do not know why this occurs.

Barrett's esophagus is a precancerous condition. This means that the cells in this section of the esophagus can become cancerous. Therefore, they need to be examined periodically for changes in their size and shape that can be the early signs of cancer. There is no cure for Barrett's esophagus. All patients with Barrett's esophagus should take a proton pump inhibitor every day to prevent any further acid damage from occurring.

Bernard's comments:

At the same time I was diagnosed with esophageal cancer, they also discovered I had Barrett's Esophagus. For the Barrett's Esophagus they were able to treat it with a new process called "Barrx." I was the first patient to have the Barrx procedure done at the Lahey Burlington facility. I had the Halo 360 done first which treated 9 centimeters of my esophagus that had Barrett's. On a second visit, I had the Halo 90 done to touch up a small area where my esophagus meets the stomach. My first check up shows that I have a normal, cancer-free, Barrett's free esophagus. I will be returning for follow up endoscopies.

21. I have difficulty swallowing food and sometimes water—what does this mean?

The esophagus, or food pipe, is a muscular tube approximately 12–15 inches in length. It propels food down its length into the stomach by a series of coordinated muscular contractions called peristalsis. Occasionally, the esophagus can spasm, or suffer from uncoordinated contractions making it difficult to swallow. Acid reflux into the esophagus is a common cause of esophageal spasms. These spasms are usually short lived and will get better with antacids and by eating slowly and by chewing your food carefully. Other times, acid can cause ulcers and scar tissue to build up in the esophagus causing a narrowing called a stricture. This can make food feel like its "sticking" on the way down. This is a more serious sign of GERD and could result in a food obstruction where food gets stuck in the esophagus for extended periods of time.

If you have these symptoms you should tell you doctor about them. Your doctor can gently stretch this area at the time of an endoscopy with a small rubber tube or balloon. The procedure is painless and very safe. Rarely, tumors of the esophagus can cause food to stick because they can grow inside the esophagus creating a partial blockage. Therefore, it is important to tell you doctor if food sticks when you have heartburn so that the appropriate tests can be ordered.

22. I often have indigestion—is it a symptom of something serious?

Indigestion is very common. Indigestion is another word for heartburn or stomach upset. Most adults have indigestion once or twice a month depending on the food they eat. Indigestion becomes more serious when it occurs several times during the week or at night. Daily heartburn or indigestion, requiring the regular use of antacids, could be a sign of GERD. If you have had regular symptoms of indigestion, let your doctor know. Most of the time these are not signs of something more serious but should be evaluated by you doctor to be sure.

PART THREE

Inflammatory Bowel Diseases (IBD)

Amy E. Barto, MD

What are Crohn's disease and ulcerative colitis?

Can I pass Crohn's disease or ulcerative colitis on to my children?

Can IBD affect parts of my body in addition to the digestive system?

Does stress or certain lifestyle choices affect IBD?

More . . .

23. What are Crohn's disease and ulcerative colitis?

Crohn's disease and **ulcerative colitis** are the two most common forms of **inflammatory bowel disease (IBD)**. Although the cause of IBD is unknown, it appears to be a result of disruption in the normal functioning of the **immune system**. The immune system is the body's natural defense system and works by protecting us against foreign substances that could potentially cause harm, such as viruses, bacteria, or even cancer. In Crohn's disease and ulcerative colitis, the immune system, for reasons that are not known, directs its attack against the gastrointestinal system, which is the digestive tract or tube in the body that runs from the mouth to the anus. As a result, in both diseases, sections of the GI tract can become chronically inflamed—red, raw, and swollen—and often accompanied by ulcers. This ongoing inflammation can lead to a variety of symptoms, including abdominal discomfort, diarrhea, rectal bleeding, fever, and weight loss.

Both diseases cover a wide spectrum of severity. Some Crohn's disease and ulcerative colitis patients become very ill and debilitated, whereas others have symptoms that are mild and easier to control. Crohn's disease and ulcerative colitis can also affect the joints, skin, and eyes and can lead to malabsorption of nutrients and weight loss, **kidney stones**, gallstones, and many other ailments. The vast majority of individuals with Crohn's disease and ulcerative colitis need to take medication regularly, and up to 70–80% of Crohn's disease patients and 25–35% of ulcerative colitis patients eventually require surgery.

Jennifer's comments:

I am all too familiar with reality of Crohn's disease. In the nearly 15 years of living with this disease, I have experienced extreme highs (symptom-free remission) and lows (debilitating pain, surgery, and recurrence) as well as everything in between. Throughout all of this I have never allowed Crohn's disease to define who I am. Rather, it is merely an aspect of my genetic makeup that I have come to accept and learned to live with.

Crohn's disease affects different people in different ways. I can only speak to my own experiences with the disease and hope that the lessons I've learned might somehow help others who are learning to manage this unpredictable (and at times, cruel) disease.

24. How do you get IBD, and is it contagious?

Crohn's disease and ulcerative colitis are considered to be types of **autoimmune** diseases. Normally, the immune system functions like a defense system, guarding our bodies against attack from foreign agents—bacteria, viruses, and parasites, to name a few. An autoimmune disease occurs when the body's immune system becomes confused and starts attacking normal organs and cells, believing that they are foreign. We don't know why this happens. One theory proposes that IBD is triggered by an infection, such as a bacteria or virus, with the inflammation continuing even though the infection has long since healed. This is known as **immune dysregulation**, or a failure of the body to regulate the immune system appropriately. Many of the drugs used to control IBD focus on modulating or suppressing the immune system. Also, some people have a genetic predisposition to develop IBD; research is ongoing in the area.

If you have IBD, it is important for you to realize that you did nothing to cause yourself to develop Crohn's disease or ulcerative colitis, and you could have done

Autoimmune

An inflammatory process in which our immune system attacks part of our own body, such as the colon in ulcerative colitis.

Immune dysregulation

Failure of the body to appropriately regulate the immune system; this lack or regulation is believed to be integral to the development of Crohn's disease and ulcerative colitis, as well as autoimmune hepatitis.

nothing to prevent it. It's not from something you ate or didn't eat. It's not from too much alcohol or coffee consumption, stress, working too hard, or from lack of sleep. We simply do not know what causes IBD. What we do know is how to diagnose it and how to treat it. Crohn's disease and ulcerative colitis are not contagious.

25. How do you know if you have Crohn's disease or ulcerative colitis, and what is the difference between the two?

From the patients' point of view, Crohn's disease and ulcerative colitis manifest with very similar symptoms. Individuals with either disorder may experience abdominal cramps, diarrhea, weight loss, intestinal bleeding, nausea, fatigue, and generalized malaise. To physicians, however, Crohn's disease and ulcerative colitis are quite different. Although both diseases can cause chronic and often lifelong intestinal inflammation, there are distinguishing features which set them apart.

Ulcerative colitis involves the colon exclusively, and almost always presents with rectal bleeding or bloody diarrhea. When the inflammation is limited to the rectum, it is called **proctitis**. In patients with proctitis, red blood coating formed stool may be the only sign of rectal inflammation. When the inflammation extends up the left side of the colon, it is referred to as **left-sided colitis**. Inflammation that extends beyond the left side of the colon is called extensive colitis, or **pancolitis**. In addition to rectal bleeding, individuals with left-sided or extensive colitis also have diarrhea and lower abdominal cramps, especially when they have to move their bowels. Patients with mild ulcerative colitis have three to six loose, urgent bowel movements per day, usually accompanied

Individuals with either disorder may experience abdominal cramps, diarrhea, weight loss, intestinal bleeding, nausea, fatigue, and generalized malaise.

Proctitis
Inflammation of the rectum.

Left-sided colitis
Ulcerative colitis involving the left side of the colon.

Pancolitis
Extensive ulcerative colitis; ulcerative colitis that extends beyond the left colon.

by red blood. Patients with moderate ulcerative colitis will have six to 10 loose, urgent, bloody bowel movements per day, along with mild loss of weight and mild anemia. Patients with more severe ulcerative colitis can have up to 15 to 20 bloody bowel movements per day, show signs of significant weight loss, and develop more severe anemia. Some individuals also describe experiencing rectal spasm, which is called **tenesmus** and is caused by intense rectal inflammation.

Unlike ulcerative colitis, which is rather predictable in its presentation, Crohn's disease is much more varied. Therefore, Crohn's disease may be more difficult to diagnose because it can be more easily confused with other disorders. Whereas ulcerative colitis involves only the colon, Crohn's disease can involve any area of the gastrointestinal tract from the mouth to the anus. Accordingly, the symptoms of Crohn's disease are mostly determined by which area is affected. Crohn's disease may simultaneously involve different areas of the gastrointestinal tract where diseased segments of intestine alternate with normal segments; ulcerative colitis always starts in the rectum and directly extends up through the colon in a continuous fashion. Crohn's disease involves the full thickness of the bowel wall; ulcerative colitis affects only the inside lining of the rectum and colon, which is called the mucosa. Crohn's disease can be complicated by abscesses and fistulas (tiny tunnel which form communications between the bowel and other organs like the bladder, skin, or anal area). These almost never appear in ulcerative colitis. Last, in Crohn's disease on occasion a certain cell called a **granuloma** appears, whereas in ulcerative colitis this particular cell is not found.

The ileum (the last part of the small intestine) is involved in about 70% of patients with Crohn's disease (in 40%

Tenesmus

Intense rectal spasm, usually due to inflammation.

Granuloma

A certain type of cell found in Crohn's disease; can also be seen in other, nongastrointestinal diseases.

of patients the ileum alone is involved, and in 30% of patients, the ileum and cecum together are involved). Patients whose Crohn's disease affects this location usually present with pain in the right lower side of the abdomen, especially after eating, and often have abdominal **distention** (bloating) as well. Diarrhea and weight loss may also be seen. At times, the ileum can become narrowed to the point that the patient can develop a blockage, or bowel obstruction.

Crohn's disease involves the colon alone in about 20% of patients. Also called Crohn's colitis, abdominal cramps and non-bloody diarrhea are usually the presenting symptoms. While ulcers in the colon are found in both Crohn's disease and ulcerative colitis, it has never been clear why little or no rectal bleeding occurs in Crohn's colitis, whereas rectal bleeding is the predominant symptom in ulcerative colitis.

In individuals whose Crohn's disease is diffusely spread throughout the small bowel, cramps, diarrhea, and weight loss usually are the major symptoms. If the disease is severe, malabsorption accompanied by significant weight loss can also be seen. Individuals whose Crohn's disease involves the stomach and duodenum experience upper abdominal pain, nausea, and vomiting as the predominant symptoms, such as they would experience if they had an ulcer.

Sometimes it can be difficult to distinguish between Crohn's disease and ulcerative colitis. This situation may occur when Crohn's disease involves the rectum and colon and represents with symptoms such like those of ulcerative colitis. In such a case, potential ways to distinguish between the two diseases include the following:

Distention

Abdominal bloating, usually from excess amounts of gas in the intestines; can be a sign of a bowel obstruction.

- Small bowel involvement—may be seen in Crohn's disease and is never seen in ulcerative colitis.

- Appearance of ulcers on colonoscopy—Crohn's disease ulcers tend to be discrete and are often very deep, whereas ulcerative colitis ulcers are more confluent and superficial.

- Biopsy—Crohn's disease has granulomas; ulcerative colitis does not.

- Fistulas and **perianal** abscesses—can be seen in Crohn's disease and are not found in ulcerative colitis.

- Blood testing—Crohn's disease is more likely to test positive for **anti-Saccharomyces cerevisiae antibody (ASCA),** whereas ulcerative colitis is more likely to test positive for **antineutrophil cytoplasmic antibody (ANCA).** Blood testing is not routinely used to distinguish Crohn's disease and ulcerative colitis, but can be used to obtain additional information when the diagnosis is in question.

It is important to keep in the back of your mind that despite our best efforts some patients originally diagnosed with ulcerative colitis may eventually learn that they have Crohn's disease. This could happen particularly after surgery is performed for ulcerative colitis, but then complications ensue, such as involvement of the small bowel after the colon is removed.

Ken's comments:

For me, this was a challenging diagnosis, and it was a couple of years before doctors were able to confirm I had ulcerative colitis. The first symptom I experienced was red blood coating formed stools when I had a bowel movement. When I first experienced these symptoms, I went to see my primary care physician, who referred me to a colorectal surgeon, who

Perianal

The adjacent area around the outside of the anus; common site for abscess and fistula formation.

Anti-Saccharomyces cerevisiae antibody (ASCA)

An antibody found in the blood that is associated with the presence of Crohn's disease.

Antineutrophil cytoplasmic antibody (ANCA)

An antibody found in the blood that is associated with the presence of ulcerative colitis.

diagnoses ulcerative colitis. However, after a flare-up about two years later, I was re-diagnosed by a gastroenterologist as having Crohn's. Later, further tests confirmed ulcerative colitis. It's easy to think that these symptoms are indicative of something less serious than ulcerative colitis or Crohn's disease, and easy to not get those symptoms checked out.

I naturally had never heard of this disease before! It's important to not take even what appear to be minor symptoms lightly, and to get checked out right away. I can't express how important it is to get early and careful diagnosis and treatment for either disease, especially because they seem to manifest in people very differently. Don't be afraid to ask your doctor questions, and do as much reading and research on IBD yourself as you can.

Jennifer's comments:

Before I was diagnosed with Crohn's, neither my parents nor I had ever heard of the disease. Therefore, we had no idea what might be causing the variety of gastrointestinal "problems" I began experiencing when I was 16. Six months later, after a battery of tests and a multitude of doctor visits, we had an answer: I had Crohn's disease. I experienced what some might consider a slow onset of Crohn's-related symptoms. My journey toward a diagnosis began with a strange taste and odor in my mouth along with a "queasy" feeling in my stomach. Although our family's dentist ruled out any obvious signs of decay or gum disease, the pain in my stomach began to worsen. Soon thereafter, my parents sought the advice of our family pediatrician, who then referred us to a gastroenterologist. At that point, I was tested for a range of disorders, including acid reflux, lactose intolerance, and a stomach ulcer. With each negative result we received back, my parents and I became increasingly frustrated; the pain I was experiencing continued to worsen and a treatment for these symptoms seemed unattainable.

At some point during those six months, the pain in my stomach became isolated in the lower right side of my abdomen. Eating became a dreaded activity (because the pain seemed to increase after meals), and diarrhea a daily occurrence. There were days that the pain—which made me feel like I was being stabbed repeatedly in the abdomen—was so excruciating that it was an effort just to get out of bed. All the while, my parents were forced to deal with the emotional heartache of not being able to help their child.

Relief came one morning in May 1992. After hobbling out of bed, unable to stand up straight because of the pain, my mom took me to the emergency room at a local hospital in an act of desperation. The doctors on call took one look at me and knew I was in bad shape. A few hours and an upper GI series later, the results were clear: I had ileitis, better known as Crohn's disease.

I spent a week in the hospital "resting" my intestinal tract. This involved hooking me up to an IV and eliminating solid foods from my diet, allowing the inflammation in the affected section of my lower intestine to subside. I went home on medications, believing the worst was behind me. Nothing could have been further from the truth

26. What tests are used to diagnose Crohn's disease and ulcerative colitis?

No one test can definitively diagnose someone as having IBD with 100% certainty. Crohn's disease and ulcerative colitis are diagnosed based upon a patient's clinical history and physical examination in combination with radiologic, endoscopic, and laboratory testing. And because each patient is an individual, not all patients undergo an identical evaluation; testing is tailored to each patient. Following is a description of some of the various tests that are used in the evaluation of IBD.

Radiology

- Abdominal X-ray: Provides a basic picture of structures and organs in the abdomen and is helpful in detecting a bowel obstruction or perforation.
- CT scan: Uses X-rays to create a more detailed look inside the body. A computed tomography (CT) scan is especially helpful in detecting an abscess and is also useful in evaluating for a bowel obstruction or perforation.
- Upper GI series/upper GI series with small bowel follow-through: Allows a close examination of the esophagus, stomach, duodenum, and small bowel. The patient must drink a chalky white liquid barium shake, and then is X-rayed as the material travels through the gastrointestinal tract. This is an excellent test to help detect strictures, fistulas, and inflammation in the stomach and small bowel. This test focuses specifically on the bowels, whereas a CT scan can also examine solid organs such as the liver and pancreas.
- Enteroclysis: Provides a detailed examination of the small bowel by passing a small tube through the nose into the stomach, and into the duodenum; barium is then introduced through the tube directly in the small bowel. This is an excellent test to help detect minor abnormalities in the lining of the small intestine that might not be seen on an upper GI series with small bowel follow-through.
- Barium enema: Allows a close examination of the rectum and colon by introducing barium through the rectum and taking X-rays as it travels through the colon. This is an excellent test to help detect strictures, inflammation, and fistulas in the colon.

- Ultrasound: Uses sound waves to examine abdominal and pelvic organs; commonly used to look for gallstones and obstruction of the bile duct.

- MRI: Uses a magnetic field to create a detailed picture of the structures and organs in the abdomen and pelvis. Magnetic resonance imaging (MRI) is especially helpful in detecting abdominal and pelvic abscesses; it can also be used to evaluate the bile duct and pancreatic duct.

- Virtual colonoscopy: A CT scan of the colon. This radiologic examination technique is still in the early stages of development but shows promise as a method to detect colon abnormalities.

Endoscopy

Endoscopy is a broad term that includes a variety of tests, including upper endoscopy and colonoscopy. Prior to a procedure, the patient receives a set of instructions describing the procedure in detail, including any preparations that may need to be made, such as stopping aspirin. All endoscopic procedures require a period of fasting beforehand. Some procedures, like colonoscopies, require colon prep. This involves flushing stool out of the colon by way of liquid laxatives and ingestion of lots of fluids. Others will tell you that the hardest part of a colonoscopy is the prep the night before.

All endoscopic procedures require a period of fasting beforehand.

Most but not all endoscopic procedures are performed under sedation, meaning that the patient arrives early for the procedure and an IV is placed in the arm. During the procedure itself, intravenous sedatives are administered to the patient directly by way of the IV line (no additional needle sticks). These medications do not make patients completely unconscious during the procedure, but rather induce a twilight state in which patients are comfortable, sleepy, and often entirely forget the procedure has happened after it is finished. Usually, patients fully wake up at the end and ask, "When are we going to get started?" More good news is the fact that the sedative medications used for endoscopies don't cause nausea and vomiting like some of the **general anesthesia** medication used for surgeries in the operating room.

Each of the following procedures (except capsule endoscopy) is performed using an endoscope (in the case of colonoscopy, the tool is called a colonoscope). An endoscope is a small, thin, flexible tube (about the width of a finger) with a light and a camera mounted on the end of the tube. This tube is then inserted through the mouth or, in the case of a colonoscope, the rectum. Endoscopes vary in length depending on the type of procedure to be performed. The duration of each procedure varies, such as 5–10 minutes for a simple upper endoscopy, and a varying amount of time between 20–60 minutes for a colonoscopy (depending on the twists and turns of each individual's colon). The physician can take a biopsy by using a set of forceps passed through a thin channel in the scope. The forceps removes a tiny piece of tissue that is then sent to a lab for examination under a microscope by a pathologist. This type of biopsy is routine and is not painful.

Potential complications of endoscopic procedures include perforation of the bowel and bleeding. These risks are very small, and the complications are correctable. Although these procedures can be anxiety provoking, many are routine and are performed by most **gastroenterologists** on a daily basis.

The following are descriptions of the individual endoscopic procedures:

General anesthesia

A form of deep sedation in which patients are given medicines to induce a state of unresponsiveness; patients under general anesthesia will not feel even painful stimuli.

Gastroenterologist

A physician who specializes in diseases of the gastrointestinal tract, liver, and pancreas.

- Upper endoscopy: After using an anesthetic spray to numb the throat, the endoscope is passed through the mouth into the esophagus, stomach, and duodenum. Although most people worry that they will "gag" on the scope, the combination of throat numbing and IV sedation allows the scope to slide down easily without discomfort. This is an excellent test to help detect ulcers, inflammation and strictures in the upper gastrointestinal (GI) tract and allows for a biopsy to be taken.

- Enteroscopy: This procedure is performed while the patient is under sedation, and is pretty much the same as the upper endoscopy just mentioned. A scope, which is longer than that of a standard upper endoscope, is passed through the mouth into the esophagus, stomach, duodenum, and jejunum. This is an excellent test to detect ulcers, inflammation, and strictures in the upper GI tract. This type of scope is not used very often, but when needed, it can be used to look deeper into the small intestine.

- Colonoscopy: The colonoscope is passed through the rectum into the colon and, sometimes, into the ileum. This is an excellent test to detect inflammation and strictures in the rectum, colon, and ileum and allows for a biopsy to be taken.

- Sigmoidoscopy: This procedure is performed with or without sedation. This is a "short" version of the colonoscopy and is used to examine the rectum and the first third (left side) of the colon.

- Proctoscopy: This procedure is performed without sedation, usually on a special tilt table that positions the patient with his or her head down and buttocks up. In this procedure, a rigid, straight, lighted tube is used to examine the rectum. Although this procedure has mostly been replaced by flexible sigmoidoscopy, it is still an excellent test to examine the rectum.

- Anoscopy: This procedure is performed without sedation, usually on a special tilt table that positions the patient similar to a proctoscopy. In this procedure, a short, straight, lighted tube is used to examine the anal canal. This is an excellent test to examine for an anal fissure or hemorrhoids.

- Capsule endoscopy: This procedure is performed without sedation. The patient swallows a large pill (about the size of a vitamin) containing a camera and wears a sensor devise around the abdomen, which is basically a Velcro belt with suspenders. The capsule passes naturally through the small intestine while transmitting video images to the sensor, which stores data that can be downloaded to a computer for your physician to watch like a movie. Because the capsule can travel where traditional endoscopes just can't reach, this test is mostly used in evaluation of patients with chronic gastrointestinal bleeding of obscure origin. Capsule endoscopy is not commonly used in the evaluation of Crohn's disease because other, simpler tests are usually more accurate in diagnosing and assessing the extent and severity of the disease. There is also a small risk in any patient that the capsule pill can become lodged in a small intestine stricture and require surgery to remove it. In patients with Crohn's disease, the chance of having a stricture is higher, which makes the chance of a capsule getting stuck much riskier.

ERCP (endoscopic retrograde cholangiopancreatography)

Procedure combining endoscopy and X-ray to evaluate the bile duct and pancreatic duct. The most common reason for performing an ERCP is the suspicion of a gallstone stuck in the bile duct.

- **ERCP** (endoscopic retrograde cholangiopancreatography): This endoscopic procedure is performed under sedation and is used to examine the bile duct and pancreatic duct. This procedure is performed for a variety of reasons, including detecting and removing gallstones which have become lodged in the bile duct, to detect tumors involving the bile duct and pancreatic duct, and to diagnose diseases like primary sclerosing cholangitis. ERCP can also be used to dilate and place **stents** across strictures in the bile duct and place stents across strictures in the bile duct and pancreatic duct.

Histology

Biopsy: Usually performed during an endoscopic procedure. A small piece of tissue from the lining of the gastrointestinal tract is removed and examined under a microscope by a pathologist. This is an outstanding test to characterize types of inflammation and detect **dysplasia** and cancer.

Laboratory Testing

Through the use of blood tests, your physician can determine whether you are anemic, malnourished, vitamin deficient, have electrolyte imbalances, or have other abnormalities that could contribute to your symptoms. Some evidence indicates that testing positive for anti-Saccharomyces cerevisiae antibody (ASCA) suggests that a patient has Crohn's disease, and testing positive for anti-neutrophil cytoplasmic antibody (ANCA) suggests that a patient has ulcerative colitis. These two laboratory tests are not routine and are not usually necessary to establish a diagnosis of Crohn's disease or ulcerative colitis.

Stool Testing

Stool tests are performed to rule out a bacterial or parasitic infection as the cause for intestinal symptoms such as diarrhea. Even individuals with long-standing IBD can get a stool infection just like any other person. Symptoms of an infection can mimic an IBD flare, and often need to be ruled out before treatments such as

Stent

Tube composed of either plastic or metal which is used to bypass a blockage in the body.

Dysplasia

A pre-malignant cellular change seen on biopsy prior to the development of cancer; can occur in the colon in ulcerative colitis or Crohn's colitis, but can also be found in other organs not related to IBD, such as cervical dysplasia (which is what a pap smear examines for) or esophageal dysplasia in Barrett's esophagus.

Stool tests are performed to rule out a bacterial or parasitic infection as the cause for intestinal symptoms such as diarrhea.

Steroid

Another name for corticosteroid; a potent anti-inflammatory drug.

Remission

The state of having no active disease; can refer to clinical remission, meaning no symptoms; endoscopic remission, meaning no disease seen endoscopically; histologic remission, meaning no active inflammation on biopsy.

steroids are used. Stool testing can also be helpful in determining causes of malabsorption.

Breath Testing

Breath testing can be performed to look for lactose intolerance and bacterial overgrowth as possible causes for your symptoms.

27. Can I be cured of IBD, or will I have it for the rest of my life?

Unfortunately, both Crohn's disease and ulcerative colitis are chronic lifelong diseases for which there currently are no cures. Fortunately, both improved diagnostic capabilities and advances in treatment have enabled the vast majority of individuals with Crohn's disease or ulcerative colitis to be treated successfully and feel healthy. The goal of anyone who treats IBD is for patients to enjoy long periods of **remission** during which they are symptom free. From time to time, you may meet someone who states that he or she once had IBD but is now "cured" and has been free of symptoms and off medication for years. Such patients are few and far between. Crohn's disease and ulcerative colitis are chronic diseases, and those with IBD should expect to remain on some form of long-term therapy to maintain control of their symptoms.

28. Can I pass Crohn's disease or ulcerative colitis on to my children?

Although it is true that both Crohn's disease and ulcerative colitis run in families, it is unlikely that you will pass it on to your children. IBD is referred to as being a familial disease in that it is not uncommon for someone with IBD to have a relative, such as an aunt, uncle, or cousin, who also has Crohn's disease or ulcerative colitis. At the same time, the majority of patients with Crohn's disease and ulcerative colitis do not have children with IBD. Crohn's disease and ulcerative colitis do have a genetic basis, and the "IBD gene" runs in families, but it is not expressed in every member of the family. Why some people with the gene develop either Crohn's disease or ulcerative colitis and others don't is unclear. For this reason, there is no recommendation to perform genetic testing on a person with IBD or that person's relatives because possessing the gene does not mean that the person will actually develop Crohn's disease or ulcerative colitis. Also, there is no way to prevent IBD even if the gene is present and expressed.

29. How do you treat IBD?

There are multiple different medications used to treat Crohn's disease and ulcerative colitis, and a variety of future medications in various stages of development. Some of these medications work best for Crohn's, some for ulcerative colitis, and some for both. Every patient with Crohn's disease and ulcerative colitis is different, and doctors need to tailor medications to each individual's situation and personal needs. In general, gastroenterologists use a "step-up" approach to treatment. This means that they will often start with more mild medications, and work their way up to more potent medications based on initial response, lack of response, or relapse of symptoms. If you are diagnosed with severe disease at the outset, you may need more potent medications right away to get their disease under control quickly.

In the first category of medications are those used to treat mild to moderate Crohn's disease and ulcerative colitis. They are called 5-ASA drugs, including Dipentum (olsalazine), Colazal (balsalazide), Asacol (mesalamine), Pentasa (mesalamine CR), and the newest drug Lialda (mesalamine). These drugs were all designed from a parent drug called sulfasalazine, which has been used for inflammatory bowel disease for many years, first introduced in the 1930's for **rheumatoid arthritis**. It is composed of a sulfa antibiotic combined with an **aminosalicylate** (also known as 5-ASA). The sulfa half is absorbed by the body and is responsible for the majority of side effects associated with sulfasalazine. The aminosalicylate remains in the colon and is the active agent responsible for suppressing inflammation. Because sulfasalazine requires colonic bacteria to split it apart in order to work, its beneficial effect is mostly limited to the colon and is less helpful in small bowel disease. And because it is a sulfa-based drug, anyone with a sulfa allergy cannot take it. Sulfasalazine also causes male infertility due to decreased sperm count, sperm motility, and abnormally shaped sperm. This side effect is fully reversible within a few months of stopping the drug. Regardless, despite these potential side effects, sulfasalazine remains an effective medication in the treatment of ulcerative colitis and Crohn's colitis and is still used commonly today.

The limitation of side effects caused by the sulfa component of sulfasalazine led to the development of the newer 5-ASA drugs listed above. These new drugs are also designed to target different sites of the gastrointestinal tract. Those that primarily target the colon, such as balsalazide (Colazal) and mesalamine (Asacol), might be prescribed for mild to moderate ulcerative colitis or Crohn's colitis. Those that target the small bowel, such as mesalamine CR (Pentasa), might be prescribed for mild to moderate Crohn's disease affecting the small bowel. Common side effects that can occur with the 5-ASA

Rheumatoid arthritis

A type of chronic joint inflammation.

Aminosalicylate

A class of drugs used in Crohn's disease and ulcerative colitis. Also known as 5-ASA.

medications include intestinal discomfort, loose stools, indigestion, and rash. Some experience hair loss with mesalamine and mesalamine CR. Rarely these medications can cause pancreatitis, and even more rarely kidney problems. A specific type of diarrhea, called secretory diarrhea, has been associated with olsalazine (Dipentum). Male infertility seen with sulfasalazine does not occur with any of these newer medications. For most people, these side effects are not severe enough to require stopping the medication, but if your symptoms of IBD seem worse on these medications, you should contact your doctor. The 5-ASA drugs, like sulfasalazine, can often take up to three weeks to become effective.

Topical, or rectal, therapy is commonly used in people with ulcerative colitis and Crohn's colitis involving the left colon and rectum. **Topical therapy** is therapy in which you apply medication directly to the tissue, much like when you apply medicated ointment to a skin rash. Individuals with IBD, especially ulcerative colitis, can be thought of as having a rash of the colon. As for the skin, applying medication directly to the inflamed tissue can be extremely effective. Topical therapy applied rectally comes in four preparations: creams and ointments (Analpram, Proctocream), which are used around and inside the anus; suppositories (Anusol, mesalamine [Canasa]), which are placed directly inside the rectum; foam (hydrocortisone acetate [Cortifoam], Proctofoam), which is squirted up into the rectum and can travel up as high as the lower sigmoid colon; and enemas ([hydrocortisone enema], Cortenema, mesalamine [Rowasa]), which are squirted into the rectum and can travel up the entire left colon.

It's normal to feel a bit of squeamishness and embarrassment about sticking something into the rectum.

Topical therapy
A type of therapy that is applied directly to tissue; commonly used in inflammation of the rectum and left colon.

Even if the entire colon is affected by colitis, it's those last 15 centimeters of inflammation involving the rectum that can cause the worst symptoms.

Corticosteroid

A potent anti-inflammatory drug.

When to start Prednisone depends upon the severity of the symptoms and the preference of both the physician and patient.

Induction of remission

Use of drug therapy to treat active symptoms and bring about a remission.

Maintenance of remission

The term used to describe the use of drug therapy to maintain a patient in remission.

However, these medications can really help a lot with feelings of urgency, rectal pain, and bleeding. Even if the entire colon is affected by colitis, it's those last 15 centimeters of inflammation involving the rectum that can cause the worst symptoms. In patients who have proctitis alone (inflammation confined to the rectum), topical therapy with cortifoam or suppositories is usually all that they need. For those with inflammation extending farther up into the colon, enemas can be used to deliver medication higher up. In many situations, combing oral medications with topical medications can increase the success of your treatment significantly.

Corticosteroids, namely Prednisone, are one of the mainstays of therapy for IBD. Prednisone is the most commonly prescribed and is used most often in individuals with moderately to severely active Crohn's disease and ulcerative colitis. Although these patients often are first treated with a less potent drug, such as a 5-ASA, others might need Prednisone right away. When to start Prednisone depends upon the severity of the symptoms and the preference of both the physician and patient. People with both Crohn's disease and ulcerative colitis who are having an active flare may require hospitalization for intravenous steroids such as hydrocortisone or solumedrol. This usually happens when Prednisone pills are not working despite higher doses. The intravenous form is stronger and goes right into the bloodstream, so it can work more quickly to bring a flare under control.

Prednisone is usually dosed at 40 to 60 milligrams a day and is often tapered slowly as symptoms improve. It can start working in as little as a several days to within one to two weeks. Prednisone has clearly been demonstrated to be effective for **induction of remission**, but it has not been shown to be beneficial for in **maintenance of remission**.

In other words, Prednisone is good at treating the acute symptoms of active Crohn's disease and ulcerative colitis, but it is not helpful as a long-term therapy.

It is important to remember that Prednisone needs to be tapered slowly over time, particularly if a person has been taking it for many months. Abrupt discontinuation can result in potentially life-threatening withdrawal symptoms. This is because while taking Prednisone, your body's adrenal glands stop producing your own natural corticosteroids, called cortisone. Slowly tapering off use of Prednisone enables the adrenal glands to wake up and restart cortisone production. So, you should not stop your Prednisone too early on your own, just because you're anxious to be rid of it. You could actually feel a lot worse if you do.

Unfortunately, Prednisone use is commonly associated with various short-term and long-term side effects, though not every individual experiences these side effects. Early side effects include insomnia, mood swings, tremulousness, acne, fluid retention, a voracious appetite, weight gain, and hyperglycemia. Long-term use has been associated with diabetes, **hypertension**, **cataracts**, **osteonecrosis** of the hip, and osteoporosis. Because of this, most gastroenterologists like to use Prednisone only when needed, and try to avoid keeping patients on it for too long.

Budesonide (Entocort) is a newer corticosteroid that has been approved only for Crohn's disease, though some physicians have used it successfully in the treatment of ulcerative colitis and other diseases such as **microscopic colitis** (see **Question 23**). Budesonide is used to treat mild to moderate Crohn's disease, and has significantly less side effects than Prednisone. Budesonide may be

Hypertension
High blood pressure.

Cataracts
A clouding of the eyes' natural lens; occurs naturally with age, but the development can be accelerated with chronic use of corticosteroids.

Osteonecrosis
Also called avascular necrosis, severe deterioration of the bone; it can be seen after long-term use of corticosteroids and is usually diagnosed by an MRI of the affected joint.

Microscopic colitis
A form of inflammatory bowel disease that can be found in the colon. Microscopic colitis causes non-bloody diarrhea.

tried prior to Prednisone, or as an alternative for those who cannot tolerate Prednisone. Budesonide is dosed as 9mg a day (three pills of 3 mg each), and requires tapering like Prednisone. The decision to use budesonide versus Prednisone varies based on an individual's situation.

Some individuals may keep flaring and requiring multiple repeat courses of corticosteroids, or, they cannot taper steroids without flaring (known as **steroid-dependent**). Still others may not respond despite high doses of steroids (known as **steroid-refractory**). In these situations, it is time to look ahead to other "steroid-sparing" medications, namely a group of medications called immuno-modulators. Two of these steroid-sparing medications are called azathioprine (Imuran) and 6-mercaptopurine (6-MP). Azathioprine is converted in the liver to 6-MP; the drugs are considered interchangeable, although the dosing is different. Unlike Prednisone, Azathioprine and 6-MP can be used to treat active symptoms, Prednisone and also maintain remission as long-term therapy. The downside to these medications is that they can take up to six to eight weeks to become effective, and most patients may require a bridge with corticosteroids until that time.

Azathioprine and 6-MP are generally well tolerated. Because these agents suppress the immune system, people are more prone to infections, most of which are minor, but some can become serious. Other side effects include bone marrow suppression in approximately 2% of patients, with a drop in the white blood cell count, and/or red blood cell count and platelets. This is easily detected with close blood laboratory monitoring. A small percentage of patients may also experience inflammation of the liver called hepatitis, inflammation of the pancreas called pancreatitis, and rare risk of **lymphoma**.

Steroid-dependent

An individual who responds to a corticosteroid, but has a flare upon tapering.

Steroid-refractory

An individual who does not have symptomatic improvement with a corticosteroid.

Lymphoma

Cancer of the lymphatic system; i.e., lymph nodes.

Understandably, many people are concerned about lymphoma. We like to reassure people that this risk is indeed rare, and that the benefits gained by controlling your IBD usually far outweigh this remote possibility. Your gastroenterologist will also order a blood test to check levels of **TPMT**, the enzyme in the body responsible for metabolizing these drugs. There are a small percentage of people do not produce enough TPMT. In these individuals, azathioprine and 6-MP need to be dosed accordingly in order to avoid a higher risk of side effects.

Another immunomodulator called methotrexate has also been used to treat Crohn's disease, but has not been shown to be effective for ulcerative colitis. It is used commonly in other illnesses such as rheumatoid **arthritis** and psoriasis. Methotrexate is used as an injection every week. An advantage of methotrexate is that it can be helpful for those with prominent **extraintestinal manifestations** of arthritis. Methotrexate is not used as commonly as azathioprine and 6-MP. It can have potentially serious but uncommon side effects, including toxicity involving the liver, lungs, and bone marrow. More common side effects include nausea, mouth sores, headaches, and hair loss.

Cyclosporine is a drug used in ulcerative colitis rather than Crohn's disease. Cyclosporine has been used for years as a vital tool to prevent rejection after organ transplantation. Intravenous cyclosporine may be used in severe cases of ulcerative colitis in hospitalized patients who have not responded to high doses of intravenous corticosteroids. Cyclosporine has various serious side effects including seizures, risk of infection, kidney failure, and high blood pressure, and should be used in a carefully monitored setting by a gastroenterologist familiar with its use. Cyclosporine can

Understandably, many people are concerned about lymphoma.

TPMT

Thiopurine methyltransferase; one of the body's enzymes responsible for breaking down the drugs azathioprine (Imuran) and 6-MP.

Arthritis

Inflammation of the joints.

Extraintestinal manifestations

Signs of IBD that are found outside of the gastrointestinal tract, hence the term "extraintestinal."

be very effective as a "rescue" therapy to avoid the need for surgery in these very sick patients. However, the possibility that surgery will be required inevitably in the future is still quite high, even months after the serious flare has resolved. It is important to remember that surgery is always an option, especially in a case like this when patients are faced with a potentially toxic medication such as cyclosporine. As always, the decision to choose medication or surgery is a deeply personal one, as there are many pros and cons for both options.

Fortunately, newer medications already in use and those on the horizon have revolutionized the treatment of Crohn's disease and ulcerative colitis. One of these medications is infliximab (Remicade). Infliximab is approved for use in Crohn's disease and ulcerative colitis, as well as other diseases such as rheumatoid arthritis and psoriasis. Infliximab is used to treat active symptoms of IBD in patients who do not respond to conventional therapy and as a maintenance drug for patients in remission. Often it is used after a patient has not responded to a trial of corticosteroids or immunomodulators like azathioprine and 6-MP; sometimes it is used initially in patients with severe disease. Infliximab is also sometimes tried in hospitalized patients with ulcerative colitis as an alternative to cyclosporine after intravenous corticosteroids have failed.

TNF

Tumor necrosis factor; this protein plays a central role in the initiation of inflammation in IBD; first described in the setting of tumors, we now know that TNF is commonly found in many inflammatory conditions.

Infliximab is a part human, part mouse antibody that is administered as an IV infusion. It's designed to attack a protein in the immune system called **TNF**-alpha, which plays a critical role in the initiation of the inflammatory process in IBD. Infliximab is usually given as three IV infusions over a six week period, followed by an infusion every eight weeks. It works rapidly, and most patients experience significant improvement in their symptoms within two weeks after the infusion; some patients feel better in just one to two days. One of the more common side effects of infliximab is the development of an allergic reaction, due largely in part to the mouse component. This is often easily recognized and treatable. Other side effects include the development of infections because, like the immunomodulators, infliximab also suppresses the immune system. Infliximab can also cause reactivation of **tuberculosis** in individuals who have previously been exposed with the tuberculosis now dormant with no signs of active symptoms (called **latent tuberculosis**). A tuberculin skin test, or PPD, can be used to make sure a person does not have latent tuberculosis which will become reactivated by infliximab use. There have also been rare reported cases of lymphoma and **malignancy** with infliximab. Those who have congestive heart failure, liver disease, and neurologic disorders such as multiple sclerosis should not use infliximab.

Adalimumab (Humira) is the newest drug recently approved for Crohn's disease (currently not **FDA** approved ulcerative colitis). Humira works like infliximab, but is fully humanized and does not contain the mouse component. Because of this, Humira has less risk of allergic side effects. Humira is administered as an injection every other week. This can be a significant advantage for people who prefer more independence and would rather not lose a half day of work for each infliximab infusion. Humira, like infliximab, is approved for active Crohn's disease in patients who have failed other drugs. Gastroenterologists are just now starting to use this drug as part of their standard therapeutic regimen. Humira may also be used for those in whom infliximab has not worked, or did not tolerate it due to allergic reaction or side effects.

Tuberculosis

An infection with Mycobacterium tuberculosis.

Latent tuberculosis

A tuberculosis infection that is dormant (inactive infection).

Malignancy

Another term for cancer.

FDA (Food and Drug Administration)

The federal agency that is primarily responsible for overseeing the nations drug approval process, and for monitoring drug safety.

Antibiotics such as ciprofloxacin and metronidazole (Flagyl) are also commonly used to treat Crohn's disease. Patients with Crohn's involving the colon and those with fistulas, perianal abscess and abdominal infection/abscess can often benefit greatly from antibiotics. Antibiotics are commonly used for other complications of IBD including C. diff colitis, and **small bowel bacterial overgrowth** which can happen after surgery involving the small intestine. Antibiotics are not used as commonly in ulcerative colitis.

Small bowel bacterial overgrowth

Abnormally large number of bacteria present in the small intestine that can lead to gas, bloating, diarrhea, and vitamin deficiencies.

30. Does having Crohn's disease or ulcerative colitis make me more likely to get cancer?

If you have ulcerative colitis, you may be at an increased risk for developing colon cancer as compared to the general population. The degree of risk is determined by how long you have had ulcerative colitis and how much of the colon is involved. The greater amount of time you have had ulcerative colitis and the greater the extent of colonic involvement, the greater the likelihood that colon cancer will develop. An additional possible risk factor is primary sclerosing cholangitis, which is a liver disorder that is associated with Crohn's disease and ulcerative colitis. Interestingly, activity of disease is not considered to be a risk factor. In other words, having severe colitis does not make you more likely to develop colon cancer and being in remission does not make you less likely. It should also be clearly stated that although individuals with ulcerative colitis are considered to be at increased risk, this is as compared to the general population in which the chance of getting colon cancer in a person's lifetime is approximately 1 in 20. Although having ulcerative colitis does place you at increased risk as compared to someone who does not have ulcerative colitis, the majority of ulcerative colitis patients will not develop colon cancer.

A direct relationship exists between the amount of time you have had ulcerative colitis and the likelihood that cancer will develop. Colon cancer complicating ulcerative colitis rarely occurs before a duration of illness of eight years. If your ulcerative colitis is limited to the left colon (left-sided colitis), risk of colon cancer occurring usually is not before 10 to 15 years duration of disease. What is not as clear is how high the risk actually is. Early studies found that the risk of colon cancer after 20 years of disease was 15% and after 30 years about 25%. More recent studies, however, show the risk at 20 years to be closer to 8%, and the risk at 30 years to be around 18%.

Another risk factor is the extent of colonic involvement. When ulcerative colitis is limited to the rectum, there does not seem to be an increased risk of cancer. The risk increases the farther up the inflammation extends into the colon and is highest when the entire colon is involved.

As with ulcerative colitis, individuals with Crohn's disease that primarily affects the colon are also considered to be at higher risk for colon cancer than the general population. The risk factors are the same—duration of disease, extent of disease, and, possibly, primary sclerosing cholangitis. The probability of developing colon cancer is the same for Crohn's disease as it is for ulcerative colitis, assuming an equal amount of colon is involved for the same length of time. However, because in Crohn's disease less of the colon is usually involved than in ulcerative colitis, the overall likelihood that a

A direct relationship exists between the amount of time you have had ulcerative colitis and the likelihood that cancer will develop.

Crohn's disease patient will develop colon cancer is less than that of an ulcerative colitis patient.

All patients with ulcerative colitis or colonic Crohn's disease should be enrolled in a surveillance program to screen for dysplasia and cancer. Dysplasia is the precursor to colon cancer in both ulcerative colitis and Crohn's disease. Because it can be diagnosed only by biopsy, patients need to undergo periodic colonoscopies to obtain these biopsies. For patients with extensive colitis, it is recommended that surveillance colonoscopy start after eight years of disease, and for left-sided colitis, after 10 to 15 years of disease. Colonoscopy with multiple biopsies should be performed every other year until year 20, at which time colonoscopy should be performed annually thereafter. If dysplasia or an adenoma is found, surveillance should be done on a more frequent basis. Individuals with Crohn's disease of the colon are at the same risk and should follow these same recommendations.

31. Is there a specific diet I should follow if I have Crohn's disease or ulcerative colitis?

Nutrition is an important part of everyday life. Good nutrition not only helps your body function at its best, but also promotes a strong immune system and a positive sense of well-being. This becomes truer for patients with Crohn's disease and ulcerative colitis. Naturally, everyone should strive to eat a healthy, balanced diet, especially those who have IBD. This said, there is no specific diet you should follow, unless certain foods have made your symptoms worse. And, along those same lines, there are no foods which have been proven to trigger a flare of IBD, or have been used with widespread success to treat the underlying inflammation associated with IBD. IBD is also not caused by a **food allergy**.

Although nothing in the diet has been shown to cause IBD, diet still does play a role in dealing with the symptoms of IBD. What you eat always has an impact on how you feel. Limiting your diet to foods that do not cause intestinal upset can make anyone feel better, even those who have illnesses other than IBD, like irritable bowel syndrome (IBS). For those with IBD, certain foods can make symptoms worse. For example, patients with Crohn's disease who have intestinal strictures (narrowing due to scarring or inflammation) are less likely to experience a bowel obstruction (blockage) if they avoid foods that are hard to digest fully, such as raw fruit and vegetables, dried fruits, nuts and berries, corn, popcorn, and less tender cuts of beef. As a rule of thumb, if it requires a lot of chewing, you probably shouldn't eat it. Food choices that have less fiber and are generally better tolerated include fish, pasta, ground beef, small pieces of chicken, thoroughly cooked vegetables, rice, potatoes, eggs, cheese (unless you are also lactose intolerant), most breads, most desserts, and soft fruits such as bananas.

People who have diarrhea from ulcerative colitis or Crohn's disease that involves the colon should avoid caffeine-containing beverages like coffee, tea, and soda (even decaf has some caffeine), because they can worsen diarrhea by "revving up" the bowels. Many patients report improvement in their IBD symptoms simply after they stop eating at fast-food restaurants.

Food allergy
Reaction of the immune system to something eaten that may result in tingling in the mouth, swelling of the throat, hives, abdominal pain, vomiting, or diarrhea.

One option for those looking for a specific diet is called the "specific carbohydrate diet," which has been proposed by some as a good diet for patients with Crohn's disease and ulcerative colitis. The specific carbohydrate diet is a grain-free, lactose-free, sucrose-free diet intended for patients with IBD and has also been suggested for patients with IBS, celiac disease, and diverticulitis. The theory behind this diet is that carbohydrates (sugars) in a normal diet act as fuel for the overgrowth of bacteria and yeast in the small intestine. This overgrowth can cause an imbalance that damages the lining of the small intestine and impairs its ability to digest and absorb all nutrients, including carbohydrates. The excess of unabsorbed carbohydrates further fuels the vicious cycle of overgrowth and imbalance. Promoters of this diet also believe that harmful toxins are produced by excess bacteria and yeast inhabiting the small intestine. By consuming only certain types of carbohydrates, people using this diet hope to eliminate bacterial and yeast overgrowth. While we do not advise any specific diet, we have seen it help in some patients. Including specific diets of any kind should be approached with an open mind, expert advice, and reasonable expectations.

Ken's comments:

I've learned over time what foods I can and can't eat. Even when my ulcerative colitis is in remission, certain foods cause cramping, gas, and general discomfort. Hot dogs are out, asparagus is a no-no, and I've pretty much cut fast food out of my diet entirely. It can be hard sometimes to avoid the foods that I know will cause me some discomfort, like at barbeques or sporting events, but with a little planning ahead I can usually get by. I always keep in mind that no matter how good that hot dog might look, do I really want to pay the price later?

Jennifer's comments:

Through what some might consider painful trial and error, I have discovered that the foods I eat (as well as those that I avoid) play a big role in how I feel. When my Crohn's disease is active, roughage of any kind—mainly raw vegetables and fruit—is the enemy. These types of food tend to significantly exacerbate the Crohn's symptoms that I might be experiencing at the time. Needless to say, I steer clear of these foods when experiencing actively flare-ups.

In contrast, when in remission, I can eat just about anything, including raw vegetables and fruit, without the painful consequences. However, for some reason, greasy, fried foods (the kind you find at popular fast-food restaurants) as well as broccoli (a former favorite of mine) send my intestinal tract into a tailspin, even on my healthiest days. As a result, I tend to avoid these types of food because the side effects, in my opinion, are not worth the few minutes of enjoyment.

Despite my good intentions to eat healthy, I have difficulty resisting some temptations. For example, my body does tolerate caffeine, but not well enough for me to avoid some mild side effects (i.e., occasional diarrhea). Rather than give up my morning coffee habit, however, I am willing to accept the consequences of my actions.

Food choices have neither triggered nor eradicated the symptoms of my Crohn's disease. However, smart dietary choices have allowed me to better control how I feel on a daily basis.

32. Can IBD affect parts of my body in addition to the digestive system?

Crohn's disease and ulcerative colitis can affect many different parts of your body. These are referred to as the extraintestinal manifestations of IBD because these effects are found outside of the gastrointestinal tract. Extraintestinal manifestations are also called **systemic** because they reflect a process involving the body as a whole, as opposed to local symptoms, which occur just in the intestinal tract. Systemic symptoms include fatigue, weight loss, anemia, and sometimes low-grade fevers. Extraintestinal manifestations can also be more localized to a specific organ. Organs that can be affected include the skin, eyes, joints, bones, kidneys, urinary tract, reproductive system, gallbladder, liver, and circulatory system. Although this list is quite long, extraintestinal manifestations do not occur in every patient. Approximately 25% of individuals with Crohn's disease and ulcerative colitis may develop one or more of the extraintestinal manifestations. Joint symptoms, such as arthritis, are the most common and are often seen together with skin and eye symptoms. Extraintestinal manifestations are found more often in individuals with ulcerative colitis or in individuals with Crohn's disease that primarily affects the colon; they are seen less often with predominantly small bowel disease.

We do not yet know what causes extraintestinal manifestations to develop, just as we do not know the cause of Crohn's disease or ulcerative colitis. The leading theory is that because IBD is believed to be a result of a defect in the immune system, this same defect could potentially lead to inflammation in other areas of the body in addition to the gastrointestinal tract. Why certain people develop extraintestinal manifestations and others do not is a mystery.

The presence of extraintestinal manifestations can provide additional clues as to the level of activity of the underlying IBD. This is because, in many cases, extraintestinal manifestations often reflect ongoing intestinal

---

Systemic

A process that involves the whole body, as opposed to a localized process; for example, fatigue is a systemic symptom, whereas lower back pain is a local symptom.

Crohn's disease and ulcerative colitis can affect many different parts of your body.

---

inflammation that may not be apparent to either you or your physician. In fact, some individuals use their extraintestinal manifestations as a signal as to when they are about to have a flare. One particular patient, for example, calls her physician and states that in a few days she will have a flare of her ulcerative colitis. She knows this because she always has an ulcerative colitis flare after she notices a certain type of skin rash.

In general, effective treatment of the underlying IBD usually leads to resolution of the extraintestinal symptoms. Some of the extraintestinal manifestations, however, run a course independent from the underlying IBD and do not improve along with improvements in the intestinal symptoms. It is also important to remember that systemic symptoms are sometimes a result of a drug-induced side effect and not from an extraintestinal manifestation.

Now you know why your doctor asks a long list of questions concerning many aspects of your overall health and does not focus just on your bowels at each visit. Crohn's disease and ulcerative colitis can affect many different areas of the body as well as the gastrointestinal tract. Indeed, at times the extraintestinal manifestations can be severe enough to overshadow a person's underlying intestinal symptoms. It is for this reason that you should inform your doctor when you are having new symptoms, even if they seem unrelated to your bowel disease

33. If I have IBD, is it safe to have a baby?

Yes, it is safe to have a baby if you have Crohn's disease or ulcerative colitis. IBD most commonly affects young men and women during their childbearing years, so naturally many individuals with IBD are concerned about whether they can safely have children. Being pregnant does not appear to pose any increased risk to women who have IBD as compared to those who do not have IBD. Nevertheless, studies have shown that women who have active, poorly controlled Crohn's disease or ulcerative colitis during pregnancy are more at risk for miscarriage, premature delivery, and stillbirth. While there are some suggestions in medical literature that even women in remission may have a very small risk for premature delivery and low birth weight, in general, women with Crohn's disease or ulcerative colitis who are in remission are at little, if any, increased risk for a pregnancy-related complication. It is important to note, however, that even for healthy women without Crohn's disease or ulcerative colitis, there is a 2–3% chance of having a complication during pregnancy. In other words, although it is safe to have a baby if you have Crohn's disease or ulcerative colitis in remission, there is still some degree of risk inherent in any pregnancy. When all is said and done, most women with Crohn's disease and ulcerative colitis have normal pregnancies and deliver healthy babies.

The best time to get pregnant is when your Crohn's disease or ulcerative colitis is in remission. If a woman is in remission at the time of conception, she is likely to remain in remission for the duration of the pregnancy. However, if that same woman were to have active IBD symptoms at the time of conception, she would be likely to continue to have active symptoms for the remainder of the pregnancy and could potentially risk the health of her unborn child. Therefore, strongly consider delaying pregnancy until your IBD has been brought under control.

A woman's overall health and fitness is also vital to having a normal pregnancy. The basic rules that apply to any pregnancy, such as not drinking or smoking, apply to pregnant women with Crohn's disease or ulcerative colitis. It is good advice to discuss with your gastroenterologist any plans for future pregnancies early on. He or she can help you plan ahead and make good decisions when the time comes. Along the same lines, you should choose an obstetrician who is experienced in caring for an expectant mother with IBD. Crohn's disease and ulcerative colitis should not interfere with your hopes of having a family.

Jennifer's comments:

After three years of marriage and more than five years in remission, my husband and I decided that we were ready to start a family. However, we were concerned that getting pregnant would pose a significant risk to my health and the health of our unborn child. My husband and I knew that getting pregnant would require a great deal of methodical planning and careful timing given my history with Crohn's. As a result, discussing my intentions to get pregnant as well as my questions and concerns with my gastroenterologist was an important first step. My doctor assured me that my chances for a normal pregnancy were no different that any other woman without IBD. However, despite the fact I had been symptom free of Crohn's for more than five years, he urged me to undergo a colonoscopy to ensure my Crohn's was not active, which would influence which medications he would keep me on. My gynecologist concurred; a colonoscopy would provide her with critical baseline information that would be used to monitor my health throughout my pregnancy.

My desire to have a pregnancy that was both safe for me and my unborn child outweighed my anxiety about the test and the results. Thankfully, we received the news we had hoped for; I was still in remission and in perfect health to have a baby. I experienced a healthy pregnancy, and remained in remission the entire time.

77

34. Does stress or certain lifestyle choices affect IBD?

Scientific evidence tells us the following:

1. Emotional stress cannot cause a person to develop Crohn's disease or ulcerative colitis.

2. Emotional stress cannot induce a flare of Crohn's disease or ulcerative colitis.

3. There is no higher incidence of major psychiatric illness in patients with Crohn's disease or ulcerative colitis than the general population.

Though stress and IBD have yet to be linked, many of our patients feel strongly that times of high stress, such as losing a loved one or starting a new job, have coincided with a flare in their IBD. This debate between science and personal experience will likely continue for a long time. Regardless, if you have IBD you should *never* feel guilty that you brought this disease upon yourself through too much stress. Certainly, being stressed out makes it a lot harder to deal with the symptoms of an IBD flare. Medications like Prednisone, which can cause mood swings, can make things even more challenging. We know that even people without IBD who are stressed or depressed can develop a variety of physical symptoms in the gastrointestinal tract, including nausea, vomiting, cramps, bloating, and/or diarrhea. This is just like getting a headache after a long day of work or from worrying. With or without IBD, your gastrointestinal tract may be more sensitive to subtle changes in your environment than you recognize. A lot of times we don't even know how stressed out we are until our bodies tell us so.

One lifestyle choice that does affect IBD is smoking. Interestingly, smoking can make Crohn's disease worse, but can actually help make ulcerative colitis better. Research is ongoing to figure out these links. Crohn's disease patients who smoke are more likely to have difficult-to-control symptoms, require more aggressive drug therapy, and have recurrence of Crohn's disease after surgery. Some have gone as far to say that quitting smoking can be as beneficial as adding a new Crohn's medication. The effects of smoking on Crohn's disease are complex and long-term and cannot be appreciated on a daily basis, such as if you quit smoking for a week to help fight a flare. On the flip side, in patients with ulcerative colitis, quitting smoking often coincides with a flare, even several years later. Nicotine treatments, such as nicotine patches and nicotine enemas, have been tried experimentally to treat ulcerative colitis, but their success has been limited by too many side effects from the nicotine itself. Regardless, ulcerative colitis should NEVER be used as an excuse to keep smoking or god forbid start smoking. The general health benefits of quitting smoking are staggering.

Alcohol consumption does not affect IBD. Of course, limiting your alcohol intake by drinking in moderation is always a good idea. Some people with or without IBD can develop intestinal symptoms like stomach irritation, bloating, and diarrhea from alcohol. The medication metronidazole (Flagyl) used to treat IBD can cause serious side effects when mixed with alcohol, including severe stomach upset, and uncontrollable nausea and vomiting.

Use of aspirin and over the counter/prescription **nonsteroidal anti-inflammatory drugs** (NSAIDs) can cause a flare of IBD in some people. There are a long list of drugs in the NSAID family, including Advil, ibuprofen, Aleve, naprosyn, naproxen, and Motrin to name a few. As a general rule, Tylenol (not an NSAID) is okay, as long as it is taken as directed.

Nonsteroidal anti-inflammatory drugs (NSAIDs)

A class of medication generally used to treat pain. All NSAIDs can cause irritation or ulcers of the gastrointestinal tract. Examples are aspirin, ibuprofen (Motrin, Advil), and naproxen (Aleve).

All in all, life-style changes can often help to improve intestinal symptoms of Crohn's disease and ulcerative colitis.

All in all, lifestyle changes can often help to improve intestinal symptoms of Crohn's disease and ulcerative colitis. As mentioned earlier, even in individuals who do not have IBD but experience intestinal symptoms with stress can benefit from stress reduction. Other lifestyle changes like healthy diet, a good old-fashioned good night's sleep, and regular exercise (with the advice of your surgeon in the immediate post-operative period) can make a difference too. However, you should always be mindful that no matter how much better you feel, lifestyle changes won't completely heal or cure the underlying disease. For this reason, you should not stop prescription medications before speaking with your physician. Regardless, lifestyle changes go a long way in improving your overall quality of life with respect to your IBD.

Ken's comments:

I can't say that times of stress have caused my ulcerative colitis to flare. Instead, stressful times result in general intestinal discomfort, as well as irritability, headaches, and a short temper. The point is, although stress doesn't necessarily make my ulcerative colitis worse, it makes me feel worse, and that can manifest in ways that aren't helped by the fact that I have ulcerative colitis. The solution? Look for ways to relieve stress. Exercise is a great outlet. Reading to my kids, listening to music, and going for long walks are all ways to reduce the stress and maintain some semblance of well-being.

35. What is microscopic colitis?

Microscopic colitis is a type of inflammatory bowel disease grouped in the same category as Crohn's disease and ulcerative colitis. Like Crohn's disease and ulcerative colitis, microscopic colitis is an autoimmune inflammatory condition. Just as in ulcerative colitis, microscopic colitis involves inflammation that affects the colon alone (which is why it is called colitis). The word microscopic comes from the fact that when a colonoscopy is performed to examine the colon, the lining of the colon often appears normal to the naked eye. Only after a tissue biopsy is performed and observed under a microscope can the inflammation be seen. There are two types of microscopic colitis, **collagenous colitis** and **lymphocytic colitis**. These two types of microscopic colitis are basically the same, except that they look somewhat different under the microscope (collagenous colitis has a thickened collagen layer in the lining of the colon, whereas lymphocytic colitis involves an excess of inflammatory cells called **lymphocytes** in the lining of the colon). Symptoms of microscopic colitis often include watery (never bloody) diarrhea, with urgency and abdominal cramping which often goes away once a bowel movement is completed. These symptoms are often mild, and similar to other illnesses such as irritable bowel syndrome.

People affected by microscopic colitis often include women ages 50–70, although lymphocytic colitis affects both men and women in this age group. Diagnosis of this disease requires a colonoscopy or sigmoidoscopy with random biopsies, which ultimately determine whether the disease is present. Treatment often consists of simple medications first, including anti-diarrheals like Lomotil, Imodium, Cholestyramine, and Pepto Bismol. For those with more moderate symptoms, drugs used to treat Crohn's disease and ulcerative colitis have been used with good success. Only in severe cases are more potent medications like Azathioprine (see **Question 29**) required, and only in the rarest cases is surgery needed for removal of the colon due to intractable and debilitating symptoms. If symptoms persist despite adequate

Collagenous colitis

A type of microscopic colitis that involves inflammation of the colon and can lead to symptoms of watery diarrhea.

Lymphocytic colitis

A type of microscopic colitis that involves inflammation of the colon and can lead to symptoms of watery diarrhea.

Lymphocyte

A type of inflammatory cell. Lymphocytes can be normally found in the blood, tissues, and organs throughout the body.

treatment, your gastroenterologist may want to check for other associated diseases such as celiac sprue.

Unlike ulcerative colitis and Crohn's disease of the colon, microscopic colitis does not increase your risk of colon cancer, and there is no need to perform more frequent colonoscopies because of it. The majority of people have mild symptoms, which resolve over the course of several months with minimal to no treatment at all. Relapse of symptoms can happen, but rarely if ever is this disease life-threatening.

36. What is ischemic colitis?

Ischemic colitis

A medical condition in which inflammation and injury of the colon/large intestine result from inadequate blood supply.

Ischemic colitis occurs when the colon suffers injury and inflammation due to a sudden disruption or decrease in its blood supply. This condition can be placed into two broad categories based on what causes the lack of blood supply. The first category involves instances that create an actual blockage, like a blood clot in the arteries or veins, and is called "occlusive disease." This can occur in a variety of circumstances, such as after surgery on major blood vessels, inflammation of small and large blood vessels, and in those who have a predisposition to forming blood clots. This can be quite serious and deserves immediate attention with surgery and/or blood thinning medications. The second category occurs due to a drop in blood supply in the absence of a blockage, almost like someone turning down the faucet delivering blood to the colon. This is commonly termed "non-occlusive disease," or more simply a "low flow" state. This second category is more common, and is the one that we will address in this question.

Ischemic colitis due to a "low flow" state is often very brief, but in some cases can persist chronically. These types of "low flow" states can occur when a person develops low blood pressure or dehydration due to surgery, significant illness including infections, medications (see below), or dialysis. Two major arteries supply blood to the colon, the superior and inferior mesenteric arteries. While these arteries have many branches to supply the vast majority of the colon, there are certain "watershed" areas that normally have an adequate blood supply, but do not have a lot of backup if the delivery of blood to the colon suddenly dips below normal. These areas are part of the left colon, including the splenic flexure (located in the left upper abdomen) and the junction of the rectum and sigmoid colon (located in the left lower abdomen).

Symptoms of ischemic colitis include small volume bloody diarrhea and cramp-y left-sided abdominal pain. The bloody diarrhea happens because the tissue of the colon suffers from the lack of oxygen-rich blood supply, becomes damaged, and sloughs off. Ischemic colitis more often happens to the elderly and very ill, but can happen in young people for no apparent reason. Extreme examples include runners who have just completed a marathon and develop bloody diarrhea due to severe dehydration. More commonly, this might occur in an elderly person who has had a stomach bug with lots of vomiting and diarrhea with inability to drink fluids and stay hydrated. Specific drugs that have been implicated in ischemic colitis include cocaine, digoxin, nonsteroidal anti-inflammatories, estrogens, alosetron, danazol, tegaserod (Zelnorm), simvastatin (Lipitor), sumatriptan (Imitrex), and diuretics. Many of these medications are commonly prescribed, and the possibility of ischemic colitis is rare, so you should not avoid them based on this potential side effect.

The diagnosis of ischemic colitis is usually made by taking a careful history to find out the possible events that may have led to the symptoms. If needed, a limited colonoscopy or flexible sigmoidoscopy to look in the left side of the colon can reveal the problem. To a gastroenterologist looking into the colon with a colonoscope, ischemic colitis generally looks different than other diseases that can have inflammation, including ulcerative colitis and infections. Ischemic colitis will often appear very swollen, with involvement of the two distinct areas of the colon as mentioned above. A biopsy of the inflamed areas can also confirm the diagnosis.

Ischemic colitis is usually short-lived, non life-threatening, and most people make a full recovery. Many people seek help in an emergency room, and are often admitted to the hospital for intravenous hydration and bowel rest. Sometimes antibiotics are used. If the injury to the colon is severe or prolonged, complications can occur such as a stricture or narrowing in the colon, as well as a perforation. These types of complications are serious and often require surgery.

37. I was told that I have diverticulosis—what is this, and is it the same thing as diverticulitis?

Benign

A non-cancerous growth.

Diverticulosis consists of tiny **benign** sac-like protrusions or outpouchings in the colon (each single sac is called a diverticulum; together as a group they are called diverticulosis). These occur in the muscular wall of the colon, often at sites that are slightly weakened by the natural penetration of small arteries. Diverticulosis is thought to be due to tension on the wall of the colon as produced by gas and stool. This condition is more often seen in westernized, industrialized countries like the United States, and is likely a consequence of our relatively low fiber American diets. Diverticulosis can happen anywhere in the colon, but in most situations it starts in the left side of the colon and may progress throughout the colon over time. These tiny pockets are most readily seen in the lining of the colon during a colonoscopy, barium enema, or CT scan. Once diverticulosis develops, it never goes away. One way to help prevent diverticulosis is to eat a high fiber diet. This helps to bulk up the stool and keeps it moving through the colon.

Diverticulosis becomes more common as we get older, affecting approximately 5% of people at age 40, 30% at age 60, and up to 65% of people age 85. Sometimes younger people can have diverticulosis, though this is less common. Diverticulosis most commonly starts in the left side of the colon, but in young people it can occur more predominantly in the right side of the colon. The vast majority of people with diverticulosis are never bothered by it, and may not know they have it unless they have been told about them after a colonoscopy. Two potential problems can happen in the setting of diverticulosis—these tiny pockets can bleed, and can become infected (called diverticulitis as discussed below). Approximately 5–15% of people with diverticulosis may develop bleeding, and 15–25% of patients may develop diverticulitis.

Once diverticulosis develops, it never goes away.

Diverticular bleeding, as mentioned above, is uncommon. Bleeding occurs as the diverticulum expands and stretches, causing injury to the small artery, which runs along side of it. Due to the very thin wall of the diverticulum pocket and the closeness of the artery, the artery can sometimes rupture into the diverticulum and cause bleeding. Symptoms usually consist of maroon stools, or bright red blood per rectum. This often happens abruptly, with a person feeling like they suddenly need to go the bathroom. They rush to the toilet, and proceed to expel a large volume of bright red blood that gushes into the bowl. Sometimes people think they've had a loose stool, but look at the toilet bowl and see only blood, or a good amount of blood mixed with a small amount of maroon stool. Rarely do people experience abdominal pain, except for some slight cramping when they are just about to move their bowels. The bloody bowel movements can occur several times in quick succession, often prompting people to rush to the emergency room.

Understandably, this type of abrupt onset rectal bleeding can be very frightening. However, the majority of people stop bleeding on their own, and rarely is the bleeding life-threatening. People are often admitted to the hospital for observation and blood transfusions. They may undergo a colonoscopy to document the existence of underlying diverticulosis as the cause of the bleeding, but usually the bleeding has already stopped and it is quite uncommon to find an actively bleeding diverticulum. Because there are usually multiple diverticulums in the colon, the gastroenterologist usually cannot tell which one was the culprit for the bleeding. Furthermore, if someone comes to the hospital with abrupt-onset painless bright red blood per rectum with a history of a previous colonoscopy showing diverticulosis, the gastroenterologist may not need to repeat a colonoscopy, but rather will observe the person in the hospital until the bleeding has stopped.

In rare cases, the bleeding persists and additional tests as performed by a radiologist can help to localize and potentially stop the bleeding. These are called a **tagged red blood cell scan** and an angiogram. Both require active bleeding to be helpful in finding the source of the

Tagged red blood cell scan

Also called a bleeding scan; a radiologic procedure done on patients who are actively bleeding internally, but the exact location of the bleeding is unclear. This test involves injection into the bloodstream of radioactively "tagged" red blood cells.

bleeding. A tagged red blood scan involves the injection into an IV of radiologically "tagged" red blood cells. These are then watched on a nuclear scan to see in which area of the colon these tagged red blood cells leak into and collect in pools. An angiogram, which requires a slightly faster pace of bleeding, involves injecting dye directly into the large arteries of the colon (through a needle stick into an artery in the neck or groin, similar to a cardiac catheterization), and watching where the dye leaks out and pools at the site of bleeding. An angiogram is additionally helpful because medications can be injected right at the site of bleeding to scar down the artery, or a plug can be inserted into the bleeding artery to do the same.

Diverticulitis involves inflammation and subsequent infection of an individual diverticulum. Lots of people mistakenly use the terms diverticulosis and diverticulitis interchangeably, but in reality these similar sounding terms mean very different things. Diverticulitis occurs when a food particle or small piece of stool gets stuck in a diverticulum, causing erosion, and damage to the inner lining. This leads to inflammation with a tiny "micro" perforation (or hole) in the colon wall, which quickly becomes infected with local bacteria, leading to a small collection of pus, or abscess, in that area of the colon. Symptoms of diverticulitis include fever and abdominal pain, most often in the left lower quadrant. Other symptoms include nausea, vomiting, diarrhea, and constipation. Rectal bleeding in association with diverticulitis is rare. A physician will usually find tenderness upon examining the belly, and there will often be an elevated white blood cell count by laboratory testing. A CT scan of the abdomen is not usually necessary to make the diagnosis, but can confirm the diagnosis by visualizing the infected area of colon along with the adjacent abscess.

Depending on how sick a person is, he or she may be admitted to the hospital for bowel rest, intravenous hydration, and intravenous antibiotics. Others may be sent home on a combination of two oral antibiotics, usually ciprofloxacin or Levofloxacin, and metronidazole. Most people get better quickly, although severe cases of diverticulitis may require immediate surgery, and rarely can result in complications including stricturing (narrowing) of the bowel, communications (or fistulas) involving other organs, and obstruction of the colon. During the recovery phase, you should stick to a low fiber diet to allow the colon to rest and heal without increasing the amount of undigested roughage moving through it.

After a bout of diverticulitis, some physicians may caution patients to avoid all nuts and popcorn, as well as foods containing seeds such as strawberries and tomatoes. The theory is that these food particles are what become lodged in a diverticulum and cause trouble. While this point is debated among physicians, the fact remains that after thousands of colonoscopies in our institution alone, no one has come across a seed or a nut lodged in a one of these diverticulum pockets. Regardless, the motto "everything in moderation" can apply to this situation as well. If someone can link his/her episode of diverticulitis to eating a large amount of, say, popcorn, then he/she would do best to avoid eating this food excessively in the future. Going crazy trying to cut out all seeds and nuts in the diet is likely not worth the effort.

One thing that a person can do to try and prevent further episodes of diverticulitis is to increase the amount of fiber in the diet. As mentioned above, this should be done ONLY after the episode of diverticulitis is fully healed. Fiber can come from many sources, including fresh fruits and vegetables, fiber-rich cereals, and fiber supplements such as Metamucil or Citrucel. There are different types of fiber supplements, including organic fiber, synthetic fiber, or a mix of both. Examples of organic fiber, including Metamucil, often can cause bloating and flatulence. If this occurs, one can switch to a more synthetic fiber supplement such as Citrucel. The same can happen with fresh fruits and vegetables, particularly cauliflower, broccoli, and beans. One should gradually increase the fiber in the diet until the body gets used to the change.

Anyone who has a bout of diverticulitis should undergo a colonoscopy to ensure that nothing else caused the inflammation in the colon, including less likely diagnoses such as Crohn's disease or colon cancer. The colonoscopy is often performed after six to eight weeks to allow for proper healing of the colon. Once the underlying diverticulosis is identified and no other lesions are found, then the gastroenterologist can be assured that diverticulitis was the likely diagnosis.

One should gradually increase the fiber in the diet until the body gets used to the change.

Surgery is sometimes offered to remove the portion of the colon containing diverticulosis to prevent further episodes of diverticulitis. This option is often discussed with people who have had recurrent bouts of diverticulitis, or those who have had a severe episode. For younger people, this issue might be brought up after a first bout of diverticulitis. Surgery is usually offered because once diverticulitis happens, repeated episodes can be more severe. And once diverticulitis happens twice, the chance of it happening again gets higher with each episode. The question of whether to undergo surgery, as well as how many repeat episodes should pass before surgery is performed needs to be decided on an individual basis.

PART FOUR

Malabsorption and Malnutrition

R. Anand Narasimhan, MD

How is food digested?

How do you know if you are not absorbing
your food and are becoming malnourished?

What are the common vitamin
and mineral deficiencies?

More . . .

38. How is food digested?

The purpose of our digestive system is to absorb important nutrients, vitamins, and minerals from food. Proteins, carbohydrates, and fats are absorbed and converted into energy we can use to perform our daily activities. The process begins in the mouth where food enters, moves to the stomach where food is broken-down. The small bowel where the broken-down food is absorbed, and ends in the colon where the byproducts of digested food are excreted.

Proteins, carbohydrates, and fats are absorbed and converted into energy we can use to perform our daily activities.

First, our teeth break down food into smaller more absorbable pieces. Chewing stimulates the production of saliva, which is made up of digestive enzymes to begin the break down of starches. Saliva also helps transfer food into the next portion of the digestive tract. As food is swallowed, it passes through a muscular tube called the esophagus. In the stomach, food is further digested by two mechanisms. First, the stomach acts as a mechanical grinder. Second, hydrochloric acid and digestive enzymes are released from the stomach to further break down food. The stomach also produces a compound called intrinsic factor to help absorb Vitamin B12.

After being processed in the stomach, food is delivered to the small intestine, where the broken down food is further digested and its nutrients absorbed. The small intestine is over 22 feet long and has three main parts—duodenum, jejunum, and ileum. The duodenum is lined with enzymes to aid in sugar digestion. Digestive juices from the liver and pancreas flow into the duodenum as well. The pancreatic secretions contain enzymes to further break down fats, proteins, and carbohydrates. The liver releases bile that aids in fat digestion. Vitamins and minerals are also absorbed in the small intestine.

After passing through many feet of the small intestine, the byproducts of food that are not absorbed enter the colon. The colon's predominant job is to reabsorb fluid. The end products of digestion make up stool and are excreted from the body through the rectum.

39. What is malabsorption, and is it the same thing as malnutrition?

Normally after food is digested (i.e., broken-down), its nutrients are absorbed into the small intestine. Malabsorption is the failure of one's body to absorb nutrients from food properly. It may occur if a disease interferes with the digestion of food or absorption of nutrients. Continued malabsorption over time can lead to **malnutrition**. Malnutrition occurs when one does not get sufficient nutrients to maintain healthy bodily functions.

Digestion can be affected by many disorders. In some cases a person has had a portion of their stomach removed during surgery. Other disorders may cause the body to produce inadequate digestive enzymes for food breakdown. In addition, lack of bile production by the liver, excess acid in the stomach, or excess bacteria in the small intestine may also interfere with digestion. Absorption of nutrients can also be affected by disorders that injure the lining of the small intestine. This may be caused by surgical removal of a portion of the intestines, infections, medications, Crohn's disease, or certain cancers.

Cystic fibrosis (CF) is an inherited disease of mucus and sweat glands that can cause malabsorption. It can affect our lungs, pancreas, liver, intestines, and sinuses. Normally, mucus is watery and keeps linings of organs

Malnutrition
Insufficient nutrients to maintain healthy bodily functions.

Cystic fibrosis (CF)
Inherited chronic disease that affects the lungs and digestive system due to a defective gene that results in the body to produce unusually thick, sticky mucus.

moist to prevent infection. In CF, an abnormal gene causes mucus to become sticky and thick. This mucus blocks tubes or ducts in the pancreas. Digestive enzymes produced in the pancreas cannot reach the small bowel and cannot absorb fats and proteins fully. Chronic inflammation of the pancreas can also cause pancreatic insufficiency, in which the pancreas is no longer able to produce digestive enzymes.

Lactose intolerance is a common disorder caused by lack of the lactase enzyme. This enzyme is necessary to break down sugar from dairy. Without it, we can have symptoms of diarrhea, cramps, and gas when drinking milk.

Celiac disease is a hereditary disorder that can result in malabsorption. It involves intolerance to gluten, a protein found in wheat, barley, and rye. In a person with celiac disease, the lining of the intestine becomes damaged and unable to absorb nutrients adequately.

Tropical sprue is a disease that also damages the lining of the small intestine. It occurs in tropical regions and is thought to be caused by an infectious agent. Fortunately, this is easily treated with antibiotics.

Whipple's disease

Rare disorder of middle-aged men in which a bacteria damages the small intestine to result in malabsorption, resulting in fever, arthritis, skin changes, and dementia.

Whipple's disease is a rare disorder that mostly affects middle-aged men. In this disorder, a bacteria damages the small intestine to result in malabsorption. Whipple's disease can also cause fever, arthritis, skin changes, and dementia.

40. How do you know if you are not absorbing your food and are becoming malnourished?

Malnutrition occurs when one does not get sufficient nutrients to maintain healthy bodily functions. It may occur due to an unbalanced diet, trouble with digestion, or difficulty with absorption. More commonly, malnourished individuals simply do not get enough calories in their diet. Their diet may lack important proteins, vitamins, or trace minerals. It can occur even with a single vitamin deficiency.

In the US, less than 1% of children are malnourished. However, malnutrition is a large problem with children in developing countries. Greater than one half of children in Asia and almost one third of children in Africa have protein-energy malnutrition. Malnutrition contributes to over half of the deaths in children in these regions. Children may present with poor weight gain and low growth percentiles. It can affect their ability to fight off disease. They may have behavioral problems like irritability, difficulty concentrating, anxiety, or permanent cognitive deficits.

Kwashiorkor and **marasmus** are two types of protein-energy malnutrition. Caloric intake is adequate in kwashiorkor, but protein intake is deficient. In marasmus, both protein and caloric intake are deficient. Those suffering from kwashiorkor have swelling or **edema**. Other changes to the body may include oral changes, abdominal swelling due to loss of muscle, damaged skin, abnormal nails, and thin, brittle hair. Those affected by protein-calorie malnutrition often have vitamin and mineral deficiencies as well. The most common deficiencies worldwide include iron, iodine, zinc, and Vitamin A.

In developed countries, inadequate food is less likely the cause of malnutrition. Instead, it is usually due to a long-standing illness. This may be due to the body's increased energy requirements to fight off disease. It may also be

Kwashiorkor

Malnutrition from inadequate protein intake often resulting in generalized swelling, loss of muscle, and increased susceptibility to infections.

Marasmus

Malnutrition from inadequate protein and caloric intake.

Edema

Excess fluid in the body that can cause swelling of extremities and abdomen.

95

due to an illness of the small bowel that affects digestion and absorption. Examples of chronic conditions include cystic fibrosis, kidney disease, cancers, heart disease, diseases that affect nerves and muscles, and inflammatory bowel disease. This may be especially seen in children who are premature, have a developmental delay, or exposure to alcohol.

If malnutrition is suspected, your doctor may order blood tests including a complete blood count, protein levels, and vitamin levels. Other tests may depend on specific symptoms.

41. What are the long-term affects of malabsorption?

Malabsorption can lead to deficiencies of all nutrients or selective deficiencies of proteins, fats, sugars, vitamins, or minerals.

Malabsorption can lead to deficiencies of all nutrients or selective deficiencies of proteins, fats, sugars, vitamins, or minerals. Symptoms (see **Table 1**) vary depending on the specific deficiency. Protein deficiency, for example, can cause swelling (edema), dry skin, and hair loss. Inadequate absorption of fat may lead to stools that are light colored, soft, bulky, and foul smelling. Inadequate absorption of sugars may cause explosive diarrhea, abdominal bloating, and flatulence.

Long term effects may include weight loss, fatigue, canker sores, delayed growth or short stature, bone and joint pain, seizures, painful skin rashes, night blindness, easy bruising, and infertility. Emotional disturbances like anxiety and depression may also occur.

Table 1 Signs and symptoms of malabsorption

Foul smelling, abnormal stools

Diarrhea

Abdominal bloating

Flatulence

Swelling

Dry skin

Hair loss

Weight loss

Fatigue

Delayed growth

42. What is celiac disease and how is it treated?

Celiac disease is a digestive disorder caused by sensitivity to gluten-containing foods. Gluten, found in wheat, barley, and rye, produces an autoimmune reaction in the small intestine that results in malabsorption. Celiac disease has other names including celiac sprue, nontropical sprue, and gluten-sensitive enteropathy.

We do not know the exact number of people that have celiac sprue, but some estimate it to be as high as two million in the United States. Many have the condition, but do not exhibit symptoms. It occurs more often in people of Western Europe and in those who have emigrated from that region. In some areas of Europe it may be as common as 1 in 100 people. If one family member is affected, there is greater chance that another member will also be affected.

As previously described (see **Question 38**), the small intestine contains many fingerlike projections called villi. These fingerlike projections help absorb nutrients and energy from the food we eat. In celiac disease, gluten produces a reaction in the body to cause inflammation and destruction of villi. This results in an inability to absorb certain nutrients. In addition to wheat, barley, and rye, gluten may also be found in many other products like cold cuts, soups, hard candies, medicines, and even in make-up.

Those diagnosed with celiac disease have varied presentations. They may have digestive symptoms like abdominal pain, gas, bloating, or diarrhea. Alternatively, they may have weight loss, fatigue, irritability, infertility, rashes, mouth sores, or seizures. Some patients have no symptoms, but may have abnormal liver tests or low red blood counts (anemia). Children that are affected often have growth deficiencies.

Patients with celiac disease produce antibodies that can be measured by blood tests. Some tests that your doctor may order include anti-endomysial, anti-tissue transglutaminase, or anti-gliadin antibodies. These are accurate tests, but a small percentage of people may still have celiac disease even if the test indicates otherwise. A small bowel sample or biopsy during an upper endoscopy (see **Question 2**) can provide additional information for diagnosis. This test requires fasting from the previous night and a ride home because of the type of sedation used. After the administration of mild sedatives, a thin flexible tube is passed through mouth into the esophagus, stomach and small intestine. In those affected, the surface of the small intestine may appear flat. A biopsy for closer inspection under a microscope would confirm this. It is important to continue eating a diet you normally would during the testing period or abnormalities may not be detected.

Over time, those with untreated celiac disease may develop other complications. Malnutrition may cause deficiencies in vitamins A, D, E, K, iron, folate, and calcium. This can result in anemia, bone disease, weight loss, and a certain type of kidney stone. Patients may also develop lactose intolerance, cancer of the small intestine, seizures, and nerve damage.

The best treatment for celiac disease is to avoid all products containing gluten. Inflammation will decrease and the small intestine will begin repairing itself within weeks. You may also need to take nutritional supplements if found to be low. Besides wheat, barley, and rye, oats as a general rule are to be avoided. Often, oats are contaminated with wheat products. Buckwheat and quinoa are gluten-free, but are often contaminated as well. It is best to meet with a dietician experienced with celiac disease to discuss which foods are safe. In general, meats, fish, poultry, dairy products, fruits, vegetables, rice, potatoes, and soy are gluten-free. Unless labeled gluten-free, breads, cereals, pasta, cookies, sauces, and gravies should also be avoided. More gluten-free products are increasingly available. Products carry better labeling and grocery stores are stocking more gluten-free products. There are many celiac websites and support groups are available which will help you manage your diet.

More gluten-free products are increasingly available.

Rarely do patients not improve while following strict dietary adherence. These patients may require medications to reduce inflammation in the small bowel and nutrition intravenously.

43. How do I know if I have lactose intolerance?

In lactose intolerance, the small intestine is unable to breakdown milk products that are consumed. In the United States, 30 to 50 million people are affected by this disorder. American Indians, African Americans, and Asian Americans are at highest risk. In addition, premature babies are at an increased risk. Lactose intolerance is also known as lactase deficiency.

Milk products contain a sugar called lactose. Lactose is made up of two smaller sugars connected to each other—glucose and galactose. In order for lactose to be digested, the connection needs to be broken by a protein or enzyme called lactase, which is normally found in the small intestine. After the connection is broken, these sugars can be absorbed into the bloodstream. Those affected may have varying amounts of the lactase enzyme, and, therefore, varying degrees of symptoms. In other words, someone with mild lactase deficiency can tolerate some amounts of lactose, while those with more severe lactase deficiency cannot tolerate any lactose products. When undigested lactose passes into the colon, it is digested by bacteria and causes symptoms. Those affected may suffer abdominal discomfort, bloating, diarrhea, cramps, and gas as soon as one half hour after lactose ingestion.

Lactose intolerance may be difficult to diagnose because similar symptoms are found in other diseases.

Lactose intolerance may be difficult to diagnose because similar symptoms are found in other diseases. If there is suspicion, your doctor may perform a hydrogen breath test. In this test, you drink liquid containing lactose. The amount of hydrogen is then measured at different intervals in your breath. Normally, there is a very low level. However, in lactase deficiency, bacteria in the colon ferment undigested lactose to produce hydrogen, which results in an elevated hydrogen level.

There are no drugs to induce your body to increase production of lactase. However, lactose intolerance can easily be controlled by diet. Most of those affected can consume small amounts of lactose products. The amount is often determined by trial and error. Also, drinking milk with meals slows the digestive process and may help symptoms. In supermarkets, look for lactose-reduced or lactose-free products. If even small amounts of lactose cause symptoms, lactase enzyme tablets and liquids are available without a prescription.

If you choose to avoid dairy products, it is important that you find calcium from other sources. Soymilk, salmon, and broccoli are just a few foods that contain calcium. In addition, you may need nutritional supplements to meet your needs.

Other hidden sources of lactose that you may not be aware of include processed breakfast cereals, bread and baked goods, soups, breakfast drinks, powdered meal replacements, and prescription medications.

44. What are the common vitamin and mineral deficiencies?

Calcium

Calcium is the most abundant mineral in our body and is stored in our bones and teeth. The remaining is found in blood, muscle, and other fluids. It serves an important function in muscle, blood vessels, and nerve function. Vitamin D helps improve calcium absorption. Alcohol can affect calcium status by reducing the intestinal absorption of calcium.

Calcium intake for adults should be at least 1000 to 1200 mg/day. Post-menopausal women usually require 1500–1800 mg/day. Most people get their calcium in products like milk, yogurt, and cheese. Other sources of calcium may include broccoli, spinach, and kale. Fortified juices, fruit drinks, tofu, and cereals are also good sources. If you do not get adequate intake from foods, you may need to take a supplement.

Folate

Folate or folic acid (the synthetic form found in supplements) is important in forming and maintaining new cells. It helps produce **Deooxynucleic acid** (DNA), which carries genetic information. Signs and symptoms of folate deficiency include diarrhea, weight loss, irritability, forgetfulness, gray hair, swollen tongue, and mouth ulcers.

Deooxynucleic acid (DNA)

A material inside cells that contains the genetic code for each specific individual.

Folate can be found in green leafy vegetables like spinach and turnip greens. Other sources include fruits, dried beans and peas, citrus fruits, wheat bran, and whole grains. Additionally, folic acid is found in enriched breads, cereals, flours, corn meal, pastas, and rice.

Those at increased risk for folate deficiency include pregnant women, alcoholics, and those with malabsorptive disorders. Adults should have 400 micrograms/day of folate. Pregnant women are at an increased risk of low birth weight infants, premature infants, and infants with neural tube defects. They should have at least 600 micrograms/day of folate.

Iron

Iron is an essential mineral found in cells. In red blood cells, it is a major component of hemoglobin, which helps carry oxygen to different parts of the body. Iron is also an important part of many proteins and enzymes that maintain good health.

Low iron levels can lead to an iron deficiency anemia. Symptoms include weakness, fatigue, and a desire to consume substances like clay or dirt. Other symptoms include slowed cognition, increased susceptibility to infection, and inflammation of the tongue. Those at risk for iron deficiency anemia include women of childbearing age, pregnant women, preterm infants, vegetarians, patients with kidney failure on dialysis, and patients with conditions that result in malabsorption of iron (celiac sprue, Crohn's disease, intestinal removal). In general, adult men and post-menopausal women lose very little iron.

Excellent sources of iron include red meats, fish, eggs, poultry, whole grains, liver, dried beans, and dried fruits. Iron from vegetables, fruits, grains, and supplements can be enhanced if eaten with meats or foods rich in vitamin C. Certain teas containing tannins and calcium can decrease iron absorption.

Males and post-menopausal females should have approximately 8 mg/day of iron. Women of childbearing age should have approximately 18 mg/day. Pregnant women and lactating women should consult a health care provider for exact amounts.

Niacin

Niacin is also known as nicotinic acid or Vitamin B3. It is a water-soluble vitamin, meaning that it dissolves in water. Excess amounts of the vitamin leave the body through urine. Thus, you need a continuous supply in the diet. Niacin is needed to convert food to energy. It is also important in maintaining the digestive system, skin, and nerves. Niacin is found in dairy products, poultry, fish, nuts, eggs, and enriched breads. Lack of niacin can cause a condition called pellagra that results in inflamed skin, digestive problems, and mental disturbances.

Vitamin A

Vitamin A is a fat-soluble vitamin also known as retinol. It is important in maintaining healthy teeth, skeletal and soft tissue, mucous membranes, skin, and eyes. It promotes good vision especially in low light. It is found in animal liver, whole milk, some fortified foods, eggs, meat, milk, cheese, cream, kidney, cod, and halibut.

Carotenoids are a form of vitamin A and are found in plant foods. Sources of beta-carotene include carrots, pumpkin, sweet potatoes, squash, cantaloupe, apricot, broccoli, and spinach. Lack of Vitamin A can lead to vision problems.

Vitamin B12

Vitamin B12 is essential in the formation of red blood cells and maintaining the nervous system. It contains cobalt and thus is also known as cobalamin. Vitamin B12 is bound to protein in food. It is released from food when in contact with acid in the stomach. It then combines with "intrinsic factor" from the stomach and is absorbed in the end of the small intestine known as the "terminal ileum."

Vitamin B12 is found in meats, poultry, eggs, milk, fish, and fortified cereals. Adults require at least 2.4 µg/day. Most people consume adequate amounts of Vitamin B12 in their diet. However, vegetarians and those with intestinal disorders that limit absorption are at risk for deficiency.

Symptoms of Vitamin B12 deficiency include fatigue, weakness, constipation, decreased appetite, weight loss, numbness and tingling in feet, difficulty maintaining balance, depression, confusion and dementia.

If you are a vegetarian or pregnant, you should consult your physician regarding supplements. In addition, those with pernicious anemia, celiac sprue, Crohn's disease, or who have had surgical removal of part of their gastro-intestinal tract may require additional supplementation. Those with a deficiency, but without symptoms usu-ally take an oral supplement. However, if patients have symptoms due to nerve damage, injections are needed.

If you are a vegetarian or pregnant, you should consult your physi-cian regarding supplements.

Vitamin C

Vitamin C is also known as ascorbic acid. It is needed to produce collagen, a component of blood vessels, tendons, ligaments, and bones. Vitamin C is also an **antioxidant**. Deficiency of Vitamin C can lead to a condition called scurvy. Symptoms include bleeding gums, dry skin, easy bruising, hair loss, and joint pains. Citrus fruits, green pep-pers, juices, strawberries, and tomatoes are good sources of Vitamin C. Adults should have at least 110 mg/day.

Antioxidant
Vitamins, minerals, and enzymes that reduce damage to cells by neutralizing free radicals.

45. Can an infection cause malabsorption?

The gastrointestinal tract normally contains the so-called "healthy bacteria." During digestion, there is a continuous coordinated activity to propel food from the beginning of the gastrointestinal tract to the end. This continuous sweeping occurs even when no food is in present. This activity also regulates the amount of bacteria in the small intestine. Disruption of this sweeping mechanism results in overgrowth of bacteria. In small bowel bacterial overgrowth or small intestinal bacterial overgrowth, there are an abnormally large number of bacteria present in the small intestine.

Symptoms of small bowel bacterial overgrowth include excess gas, bloating, diarrhea, and abdominal pain. If severe, it may interfere with digestion and cause a deficiency of certain vitamins or minerals. Severe weight loss may also result.

There are many different causes of bacterial overgrowth (**Table 2**).

Tiny muscles within the intestine are responsible for a coordinated sweeping. Diabetes can damage the nerves that control these muscles. In scleroderma, the small bowel may become stiff and fibrotic. Blockage or obstruction of the intestine interrupts passage of bacteria through the small intestine. Previous surgeries and Crohn's disease can also predispose to blockage. Outpouchings or diverticulae of the small intestine are also areas where bacteria can multiply and overgrow.

Table 2 Causes of small bowel bacterial overgrowth

Intestinal obstruction

Small bowel diverticula

Intestinal surgery

Crohn's disease

Cancer

Radiation

Tuberculosis

Small bowel bacterial overgrowth can be diagnosed at your doctor's office by a hydrogen breath test. Most sugars and carbohydrates are digested in the small intestine. Bacteria in the colon produce gas (hydrogen, carbon dioxide, methane) after breaking-down the remaining undigested sugars and carbohydrates that reach it. These gases are absorbed through the colonic wall and enter the bloodstream where they are exhaled through the lungs. In the hydrogen breath test, samples of breath are analyzed for hydrogen after ingesting a sugar (lactulose or glucose). In normal patients, if lactulose is used, only one peak of hydrogen gas should be present in the breath when sugar reaches the colon. In small bowel bacterial overgrowth, two peaks of hydrogen gas are present—one from the small intestine and one in the colon. The hydrogen breath test will diagnose only 60% of small bowel bacterial overgrowth.

Treating the underlying cause of small bowel bacterial overgrowth may improve symptoms. In addition, oral probiotics or antibiotics may be beneficial. Probiotics are bacteria that, when ingested, provide a health benefit. Your doctor may also provide a course of antibiotics including levofloxacin, ciprofloxacin, norfloxacin, neomycin, metronidazole, amoxicillin-clavulanate, or rifaximin for seven to ten days. If the condition recurs, rotating antibiotics may be used.

46. What is short bowel syndrome?

The small bowel has a significant role in nutrient absorption. **Short bowel syndrome** is a condition due to loss of a significant amount of small intestine and causes malnourishment due to inadequate absorption of water, nutrients, and vitamins. This may be due to surgery or diseases that affect the small intestine's function. The

Short bowel syndrome

Condition due to loss of a significant amount of small intestine from surgery or certain diseases causing malnourishment from inadequate absorption.

most common cause is Crohn's disease. In this disorder, inflammation can occur anywhere in the gastrointestinal tract, including the small intestine. Other causes include abdominal trauma, twisting of the bowel (volvulus), and a condition in children called necrotizing enterocolitis. This results in impaired intestinal blood flow and leads to dead bowel that needs to be surgically removed. Intestinal gastric bypass surgery for weight loss may cause short bowel syndrome, although most obesity operations do not lead to this syndrome.

One of the most common symptoms of short bowel syndrome is diarrhea. Other gastrointestinal symptoms include oily and foul smelling stools, heartburn, abdominal cramping, bloating, and food sensitivities. Other parts of the body can be affected, resulting in weight loss, fatigue, bacterial infections, anemia, and dehydration.

Treatment may require special diets and vitamin and mineral supplements. Nutrition regimens vary depending on severity of condition and ability of remaining intestine to absorb nutrients. Sometimes, IV nutrition called **total parenteral nutrition** (TPN) is needed. To treat diarrhea, anti-diarrheals, antacids, antibiotics, and pancreatic enzyme supplements may be prescribed.

Total parenteral nutrition (TPN)

Nutrition solution containing salts, sugars, and fats that is given intravenously for patients who cannot eat or cannot absorb enough nutrients by eating.

Body mass index (BMI)

Measure of body fat calculated directly from height and weight; used as a screening tool to identify weight problems in adults.

47. What is the body mass index (BMI) and how is it calculated?

Body mass index (BMI) is a measure of body fat calculated directly from height and weight. It is used as a screening tool to identify possible weight problems in adults. If elevated, other tests can be performed to calculate a more exact percentage of body fat. This may include skin fold thickness measurements, bioelectrical impedance, underwater weighing, and dual energy X-ray absorptiometry (DXA).

The BMI categories include underweight (<18.5), normal weight (18.5–24.9), overweight (25–29.9), and obesity (>30). You can calculate your body mass index using a simple calculation and without expensive equipment. In the metric system, the formula for BMI is weight in kilograms divided by height in meters squared. You may also calculate BMI using weight in pounds divided by height in inches squared and multiplying by a conversion factor of 703.

In general, BMI calculation is a fairly accurate measure of body fat, but there are some exceptions. It may overestimate body fat in athletes and those who have a muscular build. It may also underestimate body fat in older persons and those who have lost muscle mass. Other factors that may distort accuracy include bone structure, gender, and ethnicity.

You can calculate your body mass index using a simple calculation and without expensive equipment.

Elevated BMI is only one risk factor to predict disease. The risk of heart disease, high blood pressure, stroke, diabetes, high cholesterol, and cancers also depend on family history and other medical conditions.

48. How do I know if I have a food allergy?

Many people believe that they have had an allergy to certain foods. However, only 2% of adults and 8% of children have a true food allergy, which is a reaction of the immune system to something that you have eaten, such as peanuts or shellfish. Much more common is **food intolerance**, which is not an immune-mediated

Food intolerance

An adverse reaction to food that does not involve the immune system.

reaction. Lactose intolerance is a good example of a food intolerance that is not an allergy.

A food allergy occurs when your immune system responds to a protein in food that it mistakenly believes is harmful. The immune system then creates antibodies against that food to protect the body. When the food is ingested again, the immune system will release large amounts of chemicals like histamine. This reaction results in symptoms that can be mild or severe. These symptoms include tingling in the mouth, swelling of the throat, hives, and wheezing; abdominal pain, vomiting, and diarrhea may also be seen.

The most common foods to trigger allergic reactions include fish, shellfish, peanuts, tree nuts, eggs, cow's milk, and soy. Tree nuts and peanuts are the leading causes of a deadly food reaction called anaphylaxis. Anaphylaxis results in shortness of breath, low blood pressure, and sometimes loss of consciousness. Common illnesses associated with food allergies include eczema and asthma.

Avoiding the food that triggers an allergic reaction is the main treatment of a food allergy. It is important to read the detailed ingredients list of each meal. Even small amounts of a certain food may trigger a response. Those with severe reactions may need to wear a medic alert bracelet stating the allergy. If it is unclear whether a food allergy is present, you may be directed to create a diet diary. This records the contents of each meal and if any symptoms occur. If certain foods suggest an allergy, additional testing by an allergist may further aid in diagnosis. One such test is a skin test in which an extract of a food is placed on the lower arm and the area is scratched with a needle. Signs of redness indicate a local allergic reaction. If a patient has very severe reactions, the skin test is avoided in favor of blood tests. Allergic type antibodies can be measured to certain foods.

For non-anaphylactic reactions, creams often improve symptoms of a skin reaction or rash. Antihistamines can be used for congestion and itching. If much swelling is present, corticosteroids like prednisone may be prescribed. In cases of severe reactions like anaphylaxis, which is a life-threatening reaction, immediate treatment with epinephrine is usually needed. Those with severe reactions carry epinephrine injection kits with them at all times.

Table 3 Common Food Allergies
Fish
Shellfish
Peanuts
Tree nuts
Eggs
Cow's milk
Soy

PART FIVE

Intestinal Infections

Kristen M. Robson, MD

What is gastroenteritis?

Who is at risk for gastroenteritis?

What can I do to protect myself from
food borne illnesses?

I am planning a vacation soon.
Am I at risk for travelers' diarrhea?

More . . .

49. What is gastroenteritis?

Gastroenteritis

An intestinal illness characterized by abdominal cramps and diarrhea; usually caused by an infection.

Gastroenteritis is an inflammation of the gastrointestinal (GI) tract (the gut or the digestive tube passing from the stomach to the rectum). Although inflammation of the digestive tract may be due to a number of factors, most often the term "gastroenteritis" refers to an infection causing inflammation of the GI tract. Gastroenteritis is also sometimes referred to as the "stomach flu," even though it is not related to influenza.

50. What are the symptoms of gastroenteritis?

The most common symptom of gastroenteritis is diarrhea. Diarrhea consists of loose watery stools or bowel movements occurring more than three times per day. When the large intestine or colon becomes inflamed, it is unable to retain fluid, which results in watery stools. Diarrhea may be accompanied by crampy abdominal pain, bloating, nausea, or an urgent need to use the bathroom. In addition to diarrhea and abdominal pain, the symptoms of gastroenteritis may also include:

- Nausea and/or vomiting
- Fever
- Unintentional weight loss
- Sweating
- Muscle aches
- Headache
- Poor appetite
- Incontinence (loss of control of bowel movements)
- Bloody stools or bowel movements

The severity of gastroenteritis can range from mild abdominal pain, stomach upset and diarrhea to severe diarrhea and vomiting for several days or longer. Typically, however, if vomiting occurs, it lasts a day or two at the beginning of the illness. Diarrhea often lasts for a few days or more before a normal bowel pattern returns.

Because of the symptoms of diarrhea and vomiting, a bout of gastroenteritis can result in dehydration. When one cannot keep liquids down because of prolonged vomiting, dehydration may develop quickly. It is important to watch for the signs of dehydration which include:

Diarrhea often lasts for a few days or more before a normal bowel pattern returns.

- Dry skin
- Dry mouth
- Urine that is darker in color
- Less frequent urination
- Excessive thirst
- Sunken eyes
- Fatigue
- Lightheadedness or dizziness

You should seek medical attention immediately if you develop any of the following symptoms, with or without diarrhea or vomiting:

- Signs of shock such as weak or rapid heartbeat (pulse); difficulty breathing; cold, pale skin or chest pain
- Signs of severe dehydration such as little urine output, dizziness, low blood pressure, rapid heartbeat or rapid breathing
- Confusion or mental status changes

51. What are the causes of gastroenteritis?

Gastroenteritis can be caused by viral, bacterial, and parasitic infections. There are many microbial organisms (germs) that can infect the gastrointestinal tract. Viral gastroenteritis is very contagious and is a very common cause of gastroenteritis in developed countries. An infected person easily spreads viruses from person to person by close contact or during food preparation. Many viruses cause diarrhea including rotavirus, norovirus, Norwalk virus, and cytomegalovirus.

Infected food (food poisoning or food borne illness) is responsible for some of the cases of gastroenteritis. Common examples of germs that cause food poisoning are Salmonella or Campylobacter (for more information on food borne illness, see **Question 6**).

Parasites can cause gastroenteritis. Parasites enter the body through food or water and settle in the gastrointestinal tract. Parasites that cause diarrhea include *Giardia lamblia, Entamoeba histolytica,* and *Cryptsporidium.*

The germs that cause gastroenteritis are most commonly spread by the following routes:

- Food
- Contaminated water
- Contact with an infected person
- Poor personal hygiene (unwashed hands, for example)
- Poorly cleaned eating utensils

52. Who is at risk for gastroenteritis?

Anyone can get gastroenteritis. Gastroenteritis can affect people of all ages and backgrounds. Individuals at higher risk include:

- Travelers
- Students living in dormitories
- Military personnel
- Children in daycare
- Any individual who has a weakened immune system because of illness (i.e., those with HIV infection), because of medication (i.e., the recipient of an organ transplant) or because of an underdeveloped immune system (i.e., infants).

People with weakened or suppressed immune systems are usually the most severely affected by a bout of gastroenteritis.

53. How is gastroenteritis treated?

Gastroenteritis generally resolves on its own. The symptoms of gastroenteritis typically resolve within a few days. The immune system clears the infection. Replacement of fluids and electrolytes (for example, sodium and potassium) is important because these substances are lost through diarrhea and vomiting that occurs with a bout of gastroenteritis. Foods and fluids that contain electrolytes and carbohydrates can help to replace nutrients. Fluid and electrolyte replacement solutions can be purchased at most grocery stores and pharmacies. The **Centers for Disease Control** (CDC) recommends oral rehydration solutions (ORS). These are available without a prescription. If fluid loss is significant, hospitalization is usually required, and nutrients and fluids can be replaced intravenously (i.e., injected directly into the vein).

If you are dehydrated, a health care professional will advise you on how much to drink. The oral rehydration solutions provide a balance of water, salt, and sugar, such

People with weakened or suppressed immune systems are usually the most severely affected by a bout of gastroenteritis.

Centers for Disease Control (CDC)

The federal facility for disease eradication, epidemiology, and education that is located in Atlanta, Georgia.

as Gatorade, Crystal Light, or Pedialyte. They are better than just drinking water alone. A small amount of sugar and salt helps with absorption of the water from the gut or intestines into the body. The oral rehydration solutions do not reduce the amount of diarrhea, but they do help to prevent or treat dehydration. It is recommended that you do not use homemade salt and sugar drinks, as the quantity of the salt and sugar has to be exact. It is best to avoid drinks that contain a lot of sugar such as undiluted fruit juices or soft drinks.

Antibiotics are not effective if the cause of gastroenteritis is a viral infection. Antidiarrheal drugs are usually not necessary and they may prolong the duration of the infection. As always, if symptoms are severe or persist, it is best to seek medical attention.

54. What is a food borne illness?

Consumption of contaminated foods or beverages is the cause of a food borne illness. Many different germs or **microbes** can contaminate foods, and thus there are many different food borne illnesses. Bacteria (or their toxins), viruses, and parasites can all cause food borne illness. Many food borne illnesses have been described. The illnesses range from upset stomach to more serious symptoms such as fever, vomiting, diarrhea, and dehydration. Since the microbe or toxin enters the body through the gastrointestinal tract, nausea, vomiting and diarrhea are common manifestations of food borne illness. Because many individuals who develop and recover from a food borne illness do not seek medical attention, many food borne illnesses are not reported. The Centers for Disease Control and Prevention (CDC) estimates that, each year, about 76 million people in the United States contract a food borne illness.

Microbe

A very tiny organism.

55. What are the most common food borne illnesses?

Table 4 Common Sources of Food Borne Illness

Source of Illness	Symptoms	Microbe
Raw and undercooked meat and poultry	Abdominal pain Nausea and vomiting	Bacteria: *Campylobacter jejuni* *E. Coli 0157:H7* *L. monocytogenes* *Salmonella*
Raw (i.e., unpasteurized) milk and dairy products such as soft cheeses	Nausea and vomiting Abdominal cramps Diarrhea Fever	Bacteria: *L. monocytogenes* *Salmonella* *Shigella* *Staphylococcus aureus* *Campylobacter jejuni*
Raw or undercooked eggs (including those found in salad dressings, cookie dough, sauces and frosting)	Nausea and vomiting Abdominal cramps Diarrhea Fever	Bacteria: *Salmonella enteriditis*
Raw or undercooked shellfish	Chills and fever Collapse	Bacteria: *Vibrio vulnificus* *Vibrio parahaemolyticus*
Improperly canned goods Improperly smoked or salted fish	Double vision Difficulty speaking, swallowing Difficultly breathing (seek medical attention immediately)	Bacteria: *C. botulinum*
Fresh produce	Diarrhea Nausea and vomiting	Bacteria: *L. monocytogenes* *Salmonella* *Shigella* *E. Coli 0157:H7* *Yersinia enterocolitica* *Viruses and parasites*
Cold foods including sandwiches, salads and bakery products Salad dressing Cake frosting Oysters Raspberries	Nausea and vomiting Diarrhea Abdominal cramps Low grade fever, chills Headache	*Virus:* *Norovirus (family Caliciviridae)*

56. How does food become contaminated?

Food may become contaminated during the growing, harvesting, processing, storing, shipping, or final preparation of food. There are many sources for food **contamination**. Raw foods are not sterile. Many food borne germs and microbes are present in healthy animals raised for food. Raw meat and poultry may become contaminated during slaughter. Fresh fruits and vegetables may be contaminated if they are washed or irrigated with water that is contaminated. Water can be contaminated by either animal manure or human sewage. Food items that are grown in soil may be contaminated during the growth or through processing and distribution.

In food processing, food borne microbes can be introduced from humans who handle the food. The unwashed hands of infected food handlers can introduce bacteria such as *Shigella* and viruses such as Hepatitis A. In the preparation of food, germs can be transferred from one food to another food by using the same utensils or cutting boards to prepare both without washing the utensil or surface in between. A fully cooked food can become re-contaminated if it comes in contact with other raw foods that contain microbes.

When food is cooked and left at room temperature for over two hours, bacteria can multiply quickly. Many bacteria need to multiply to a larger number before the food can cause illness. If food is left at room temperature, one bacterium can multiply so rapidly that food left out overnight can be highly infectious by the next day. If food is refrigerated promptly, bacteria cannot multiply.

Contamination

The process of rendering impure or unsuitable by contact; mixture or introduction of an undesirable element.

When food is cooked and left at room temperature for over two hours, bacteria can multiply quickly.

Freezing foods slows or stops bacterial growth, but freezing does not destroy bacteria. When food is thawed, bacteria or germs can become reactivated and the food still needs to be cooked thoroughly. Refrigeration may slow the growth of some bacteria but thorough cooking is also needed to destroy it. High salt, high sugar, or high acid levels also prevent bacterial growth, and these substances are traditionally used as preservatives in certain salted meats, jams, and pickled vegetables.

If food is heated to an internal temperature above 160° F or 71° C, this is generally sufficient to kill parasites, viruses, or bacteria, except for the *Clostridium* bacteria. *Clostridium* bacteria produce a heat resistant form called a spore. *Clostridium* spores are killed only at temperatures above boiling. Canned foods must be cooked to a high temperature under pressure as part of the canning process for this reason.

57. What can I do to protect myself from food borne illnesses?

Most cases of food borne illness can be prevented through proper cooking and processing of food. These simple precautions can reduce the risk of food borne illness:

- *Cook* meat, poultry and eggs thoroughly. Use a thermometer to measure the internal temperature of meat. For example, ground beef should be cooked to an internal temperature of 160° F. Eggs should be cooked such that the yolk is firm. Foods are properly cooked only when they are heated long enough and at the necessary temperature to kill harmful bacteria.

- *Clean.* Food handlers should always wash their hands before touching food and after using the bathroom, handling pets, as well as handling raw meat, poultry, fish, or eggs. Produce, fresh fruits, and vegetables should be cleansed in tap water to remove visible dirt. The outermost leaves of lettuce and cabbage should be discarded.

- *Separate.* Wash all utensils, knives, and cutting boards thoroughly after they have been in contact with raw meat or poultry. Cooked meat should be placed on a clean plate or platter and should never be placed on the original one that held the raw meat.

- *Chill.* Refrigerate foods promptly. If a prepared food has been at room temperature for more than two hours, it may not be safe to eat. Refrigerators should be set at 40° F or lower and the freezer should be set at 0° F. It is ideal to a divide large amount of food into smaller containers for quick cooling. Do not pack the refrigerator. Cool air must circulate to keep foods safe. Never defrost food at room temperature (i.e., on the kitchen counter). Use the refrigerator or cold running tap water.

- *Keep cold foods cold and hot foods hot.*

If a food borne illness is suspected, it is always advisable to report this to the local health department. Often concerned citizens are the first to report a suspected outbreak of a food borne illness. For more information and guidelines, please see:

- U.S. Drug and Food Administration: *www.fda.gov*
- Centers for Disease Control and Prevention: *www.cdc.gov*

- Partnership for Food Safety Education:
  www.fightbac.org
- U.S. Department of Agriculture:
  www.usda.gov
- U.S. Department of Health and Human Services:
  www.os.dhhs.gov

58. I am planning a vacation soon. Am I at risk for travelers' diarrhea?

Travelers' diarrhea is the most common illness among travelers to developing countries. 40–60% of people traveling to any part of the developing world may develop diarrhea. Although an attack of travelers' diarrhea almost always resolves on its own, dehydration may occur and may be more serious than the diarrhea itself.

Bacteria, viruses, and parasites can all cause diarrheal illness in travelers, but in most areas, the majority of illnesses are caused by bacteria. The organisms (i.e., germs) are typically transmitted by food and water. The most common bacteria is enterotoxigenic *Escherichia coli* (ETEC).

The risk of developing travelers' diarrhea depends on the travel destination. There are three levels of risk that correspond to the geographic region.

- Low risk (less than 10%): Northern Europe, Australia, New Zealand, the United States, Canada, and Singapore
- Moderate risk (10–20%): Caribbean Islands, South Africa, and countries bordering the Mediterranean Ocean, including Israel

- High risk (greater than 30%): Asia (with the exception of Singapore), Africa (outside of South Africa), South and Central America, and Mexico.
- The following organisms can be responsible for travelers' diarrhea (note: this is not a comprehensive list but includes several examples):

Bacteria

1. Enterotoxigenic *Escherichia coli*
2. Enteroaggregative *Escherichia coli*
3. *Campylobacter jejuni*
4. *Salmonella* species
5. *Vibrio parahaemolyticus* or *vibrio cholera*

Viruses

1. *Rotavirus*
2. *Norovirus*

Parasites

1. *Giardia lamblia*
2. *Cryptosporidium parvum*
3. *Cyclospora cayetanensis*

The typical case of travelers' diarrhea may occur between four days and two weeks after arrival. The symptoms can vary depending on which organism or germ is responsible for the infection. Symptoms may include any of the following: watery diarrhea, fatigue, loss of appetite, abdominal cramping, nausea, vomiting, and low-grade fever.

There are several strategies that travelers can utilize to reduce their risk of acquiring a diarrheal illness.

59. What can I do to prevent travelers' diarrhea?

There are several strategies that travelers can utilize to reduce their risk of acquiring a diarrheal illness. The Infectious Diseases Society of America (a group of physicians and health care professionals who are experts in the diagnosis and treatment of infections) has established guidelines on advice for travelers, including the strategies listed below.

- *Be careful in choosing what you eat and drink.* There are many factors that contribute to the transmission of organisms or germs though food and water. Freezing does not kill organisms that cause diarrhea. Ice is unsafe unless it has been made with filtered or boiled water. Alcohol does not sterilize water. Carbonated water is usually safe (check to see that the water or soft drink has been sufficiently carbonated when the bottle is opened). The ingredients in chicken or fruit salads and lettuce may have been improperly cleansed or may have not been refrigerated properly and these foods are generally considered unsafe. Condiments can frequently become contaminated. Bottled drinks should be consumed from the bottle with a straw and should be consumed without ice. Fruits that are peeled just prior to eating are considered safe.

- *Consider the water supply and use purification measures if necessary.* Bottled water and soft drinks are generally available to most travelers. Hot tea and coffee are usually safe alternatives to bottled water. For those who are traveling to more remote areas, water purification may be necessary. Water can be purified in a number of ways:

  1. Boiling for three minutes followed by cooling to room temperature
  2. At camping or wilderness supply stores, you can find compact water filters, which use iodine in the filter to remove parasites and kill viruses and bacteria.

- *Consider oral antibiotics as prevention only if the potential benefit outweighs the risk.* Antibiotics can prevent most cases of travelers' diarrhea but they are not routinely recommended unless the potential diarrhea and/

or dehydration could result in severe complications of an underlying medical illness, such as congestive heart failure. In other words, the benefit of the antibiotic must outweigh its risk. Antibiotics can have multiple side effects including allergic reaction, sun sensitivity, yeast (fungal) infections, and altering the normal numbers of good bacteria that live in or colonize the large intestine. When the usual good bacteria counts in the large intestine are altered, this can increase the risk of development of a potentially serious infection called *Clostridium difficile* colitis or *C. diff* colitis. *C. diff* colitis can present as a mild or severe diarrheal illness that usually requires antibiotic treatment. If severe, *C. diff* colitis may require hospitalization as well. Rare complications of severe *C. diff* colitis include perforation (i.e., a hole in the wall of the large intestine) and infrequently, surgical removal of the colon is necessary.

Travelers who may consider the use of antibiotics to prevent diarrhea include those with chronic inflammatory bowel disease such as ulcerative colitis or Crohn's disease, those with significant heart or kidney disease or those with suppressed immune systems such as individuals with HIV infection, or recipients of an organ transplant.

60. What is the treatment for travelers' diarrhea?

Travelers' diarrhea can be managed with one or more of the following:

- Fluid replacement
- Antibiotics
- Agents that slow the motility or movement of the bowels and thus decrease the episodes of diarrhea

INTESTINAL INFECTIONS

Fluid Replacement

The most important treatment for travelers' diarrhea is fluid replacement since the most significant risk is dehydration. For cases of mild diarrhea, broth, diluted fruit juice, or similar fluids may be used. For cases of severe diarrhea, an oral rehydration solution should be used. An oral rehydration solution replaces the needed electrolytes in precise concentrations. In most cases of diarrhea, the intestine can still absorb glucose (sugar) that is linked to a salt water solution. Oral rehydration solution is available in most pharmacies and grocery stores. The composition of fluids that are used as sport drinks for sweat replacement is not similar to oral rehydration solution. For mild cases of diarrhea however, oral rehydration solution is not absolutely necessary and generic fluids can be used.

Antibiotics

Antibiotic treatment is generally needed in those who develop moderate to severe diarrhea (greater than four watery stools per day) or fever. Some travelers may be given a prescription for antibiotics that can be taken if diarrhea develops. Medical attention may be necessary for individuals who develop high fever, abdominal pain, bloody diarrhea, or vomiting. The most commonly prescribed antibiotic for travelers' diarrhea is ciprofloxacin (500 mg by mouth twice daily), given for one or two days. Treatment with ciprofloxacin or a related antibiotic (i.e., quinolone) will lead to resolution of diarrheal symptoms in the majority of travelers within one day.

Antimotility Agents

Antimotility agents such as loperamide (Imodium) are often used to treat the symptom of diarrhea. They do not treat the underlying cause of the diarrhea. There is concern that antimotility agents may prolong the diarrheal illness. If there is any sign of bloody diarrhea or abdominal pain, antimotility agents should NOT be used. Even though the diarrhea may improve with the use of antimotility agents, it remains important to stay adequately hydrated. For most cases of travelers' diarrhea, antimotility agents are not recommended.

61. How do I know if I have a parasite?

An infection caused by a parasite can be diagnosed in a number of ways.

An infection caused by a parasite can be diagnosed in a number of ways. The type of test will depend on the signs and symptoms, medical history, and travel history of the patient. The following tests are available to help in the diagnosis of parasitic diseases:

1. *Stool examination for parasites (called an ova and parasite or O&P test)*

   This test can be used to determine if a parasite is the cause of diarrhea, cramping, gas, and other abdominal symptoms. Because the shedding of parasites is intermittent, the Centers for Disease Control (CDC) recommends that three stool samples, collected at least 24 hours apart, be examined. For most cases of diarrhea caused by a parasite, stool culture or testing is not needed, as the symptoms and illness typically are limited to a few days. If symptoms persist or if there are risk factors for parasitic illness such as travel to a mountainous region or exposure to infants at a dare care center, then stool testing may be indicated. The stool testing looks for the ova (eggs) or the parasite.

2. *Endoscopy*

Endoscopy can be used to look for parasites that cause diarrhea, abdominal pain or cramping, gas, or other gastrointestinal symptoms. This test is an invasive procedure in which a tube is inserted into the mouth or rectum so that the lining of the intestine can be directly examined. During this exam, biopsies can be obtained and specimens can be obtained for culture if needed.

3. *Blood tests*

Testing the blood can identify some parasitic infections. Blood tests look for a specific parasite. One type of blood test (called a serology) looks for antibodies that are produced when the immune system of the infected individual is trying to fight off the parasite. Some parasitic diseases, such as malaria, can be diagnosed by looking at a blood smear under the microscope. This test is done by placing a drop of blood on a microscope slide. The slide is then examined under a microscope.

4. *X-rays*

In some cases, an X-ray such as a computerized axial tomography (CAT) scan or a magnetic resonance imaging (MRI) scan can be helpful in diagnosing parasitic diseases.

For more information on parasitic illness, see the Website for the Centers for Disease Control, *www.cdc.gov.*

PART SIX

Gastrointestinal Cancer

Ann Marie Joyce, MD

When should I have a colonoscopy?

I've had heartburn for many years—am I at risk of developing esophageal cancer?

How do you diagnose cancer of the liver?

More . . .

62. How do I know if I have colon cancer?

Colon cancer is the fourth most common type of cancer. There were about 145,000 new cases of colorectal cancer diagnosed in 2005. The risk of developing colon cancer in your lifetime is 6%, which means that 6 people out of 100 people will develop cancer of the colon. There is an increased risk of developing colon cancer in certain groups of people. Patients that are at increased risk include patients with a family history of colon cancer, a familial polyp syndrome, or inflammatory bowel disease.

Patients with colon cancer may have a variety of different complaints, although some individuals may not have any symptoms. Some people may have blood in the stool. Bright red blood can indicate bleeding on the left side of the colon whereas darker blood suggests bleeding from the right side of the colon. Many patients will not see blood in the stool, but a tiny amount may be present. This tiny amount of blood can be detected using stool cards done at the time of rectal examination or stool cards that are taken home. This is called occult bleeding. Stool cards are effective means of colorectal screening. A positive stool card indicating the presence of blood requires a colon evaluation. This bleeding can lead to iron deficiency anemia, which is low red blood cell count. A complete blood count is a blood test that can detect anemia; it is usually performed at the time of an annual physical examination.

Some patients present with a change in bowel movements. Most people have a regular bowel pattern ranging from three bowel movements a day to one bowel movement every three days. A change in this pattern can indicate colon cancer. Pencil-shaped bowel movements have often been considered to be a strong indication of colon cancer, but it is usually just a sign of constipation.

Other less common complaints are a lack of appetite or unexplained weight loss. These two symptoms may be associated with a variety of other conditions such as stomach cancer, thyroid problems, diabetes mellitus, or depression.

There are also a group of patients that have no symptoms related to colon cancer and therefore it is recommended that all people over the age of 50 should be screened for colon cancer.

63. When should I have a colonoscopy?

Colonoscopy has become the standard of care for colon cancer screening. Colonoscopy is an effective means to evaluate the colon and has been shown to prevent colon cancer. The colonoscope is a flexible tube with a camera and light that can be maneuvered through the colon. If you are scheduled for a colonoscopy it is important to be familiar with the instructions. You should decrease your fiber intake about one week prior to the procedure. If you are prone to constipation you should try to have daily bowel movements the week prior to the procedure.

The day before the colonoscopy you should only take clear liquids. Clear liquids are defined as anything that you can see through. Examples of clear liquids include Jell-O, broth, juice, and coffee and tea without milk. You should drink plenty of fluids the day prior to the procedure. In the evening prior to the procedure you should take the preparation. The preparations vary from endoscopy units. It is usually a laxative with a large quantity of liquid. Within a few hours of taking the preparation you will begin to have bowel movements. You will probably have several bowel movements throughout the night. A good preparation is defined by liquid bowel movements that are very light in color (sometimes similar to the color of urine). A lot of patients feel nauseated with the preparation. To avoid feeling nauseated, you should chill the preparation. If you feel nauseated while drinking the preparation, then slowly drink it. Remember, you should do your best to complete the entire drink. You should have nothing to eat or drink six hours prior to the procedure. You should arrive at the endoscopy department at the assigned time. You will need to have a ride to take you home. You should bring a list of your medications and drug allergies with you.

In the endoscopy unit, you will change into a hospital gown. An intravenous (IV) line will be placed in order to give you sedation. The procedure will be explained to you in detail and you will sign a permission sheet (i.e., consent form). In the procedure room, you will be attached to heart and respiratory monitors and given supplemental oxygen through nasal prongs. Most colonoscopies are performed with conscious sedation, which is a type of mild anesthesia. During the procedure you are in a twilight zone. You are breathing on your own and you may hear voices around you. For the most part you are unaware of the procedure taking place.

The doctor starts with a rectal examination. The colonoscope is inserted into the rectum and maneuvered to the cecum, which is the part of the colon where it meets the small bowel. As the colonoscope is inserted into the colon, you may feel some cramping. The colon is insufflated with air so the cramping may resemble gas pains. Upon reaching the cecum, the camera will be withdrawn and the lining of the colon carefully examined. Polyps (growths within the colon) can be removed at this time. Biopsies can also be taken. After the procedure is completed, you will return to the recovery room. You may feel sleepy. You may experience bloating. It is important to release the excess air that was instilled during the procedure.

After leaving the endoscopy unit, you are not permitted to drive. You will not be able to drive or operate heavy machinery that day. You may feel fine, but the medications stay within your system for the remainder of the day. If you experience abdominal pain, bleeding, fever, chills, nausea, or vomiting within 24 hours after the procedure then you should contact your doctor or go to the nearest emergency room.

Colonoscopy is a safe procedure, but as with all procedures, there are risks involved. Complications occur in about 1 in 1000 patients. Some of the complications include bleeding requiring a blood transfusion, perforation (hole or tear) that can result in surgery, or a reaction to the medication. It is felt that the benefits of the procedure far outweigh these risks.

As mentioned in **Question 62**, patients can have colon cancer without symptoms. Therefore, current guidelines recommend that every individual should be screened for colon cancer. The average risk patient is defined as someone without symptoms, no family or personal history of colon cancer or colon polyps, and no inflammatory bowel disease. An average risk person (the majority

The average risk patient is defined as someone without symptoms, no family or personal history of colon cancer or colon polyps, and no inflammatory bowel disease.

of people) should have the first colonoscopy performed at 50. In patients with a family history of colon cancer or colon polyps in first relatives 60 or younger (first degree is defined as parent, sibling or child), screening should start at 40 years or ten years younger than the affected relative. The frequency or screening is determined by the individual's personal risk of developing colon cancer. For an average risk person, the current guidelines recommend a colonoscopy every 10 years. For a person with a family history of colon cancer, a colonoscopy every 5 years is recommended.

After your first colonoscopy, your risk of developing colon cancer is re-evaluated. If you have no polyps and you have no risk factors for developing colon cancer, then you can wait 10 years until your next colonoscopy. If you have a polyp, then your risk of developing colon cancer may be increased. What is a polyp? There are two major types of polyps found in the colon. The first type is a hyperplastic polyp, which has no potential in developing into a colon cancer. Adenomas are the second type of polyp. Adenomas have the potential to grow into a colon cancer over a 5 to 15 year period. The goal of a colonoscopy is to remove polyps to prevent colon cancer. All polyps are removed at the time of a colonoscopy. The polyps are then sent to the pathology laboratory in order to determine the type of polyp. Once adenomatous polyps are detected, the risk of colon cancer is increased and therefore your next colonoscopy should be performed in three to five years. Usually larger, numerous polyps require repeat procedure in three years. There are certain circumstances, such as change in personal or family history, which may influence date of the next colonoscopy.

64. What is a virtual colonoscopy?

A virtual colonoscopy is a special CT scan of the colon. A CT scan is an X-ray that displays pictures of the body as if it was sliced like a loaf of bread. The slices can be as small as 3 mm. Once the CT scan has been performed, a computer program processes the pictures from a two-dimensional to a three dimensional format. CT scans are performed for a variety of different reasons, but not all CT scans are the same. The virtual colonoscopy is a CT scan that has been used as a tool for screening for colon cancer. You still need to clean out your colon with a prescription laxative similar to a colonoscopy. The CT scan is usually done in the radiology department. It takes about 10 minutes. You will be asked to lie on your back on the table. A tube is placed into the rectum so that air can be pumped into the colon. This allows improved imaging of the colon. During the examination you will be asked to hold your breath to avoid distortion of the images. You will be asked then to turn onto your stomach and the scan will be repeated. You will not be given sedation for the CT scan. Therefore, you do not need to take the day off work or need a ride home.

Virtual colonoscopy has the potential to be a good screening test. Studies have shown that some patients prefer the virtual colonoscopy to an actual colonoscopy. The procedure does not require sedation so that you can drive yourself home and don't have to miss a day of work. The procedure also takes less time to perform. Virtual colonoscopy is quite accurate for detecting polyps greater than 6mm. Larger polyps are usually the polyps that are more dangerous (i.e., higher risk of cancer). At this point, virtual colonoscopy has not replaced the standard colonoscopy. What are the disadvantages of virtual colonoscopy? You must still take a preparation to clean out the colon similar to the preparation prior to standard colonoscopy. Similar to a standard colonoscopy, air is instilled into the colon to inflate the colon. This can be an uncomfortable part of the both procedures. While sedation is given at the time of a colonoscopy to ease this cramping, no sedation is given to the patient at the time of a virtual colonoscopy. The virtual colonoscopy is an X-ray and exposes the patient to radiation. Insurance companies do not cover the procedure. While the virtual colonoscopy can detect larger polyps (>6 mm) and masses within the colon, it is not reliable to detect smaller polyps. And there is a very small risk of precancerous cells in smaller polyps. If the virtual colonoscopy demonstrates an abnormality, then a follow up colonoscopy will still be required to remove the polyp.

Someday virtual colonoscopy may become the standard of care for colon cancer screening. The future of virtual colonoscopy includes better imaging, improved acceptance by insurance companies, and a prepless procedure.

65. I read that there is a tiny camera that you can swallow to examine the digestive tract—can I do this instead of a colonoscopy?

There is a tiny camera that is available to examine the digestive system. Developed in the late 1990s, the camera is the size of a multivitamin. Currently there are two cameras that are approved for use by the food and drug administration (FDA). There is one capsule that can evaluate the esophagus (the food pipe) and there is another capsule that can examine the small bowel. The small bowel is the area of the digestive tract between the stomach and the colon (or large intestine). It is about 20 feet in length. While swallowing a capsule to examine the colon is an attractive alternative to a colonoscopy, currently this technology exists only in the developmental stage.

In addition to the capsule, there are two more traditional ways to examine the esophagus. The oldest test is an esophagogram. This is an X-ray test in which the patient drinks barium (a white chalky material) and X-rays are taken of the esophagus. The second type of examination is an upper endoscopy. This is a procedure where a flexible tube with a camera is inserted through the mouth, into the esophagus, and then the stomach and first portion of the small intestine. Upper endoscopy is usually performed with sedation. The third type of examination and the most recent is with a capsule called the esocapsule, or esophagus capsule. The examination takes about 15 minutes. After going through the esophagus, the capsule travels through the remainder of the digestive system and eventually passed with a bowel movement. Most people do not see the capsule in the toilet bowl. The pictures of the esophagus are captured on a data recorder, which the patient wears during the procedure. The images are downloaded to a computer and reviewed as a short movie. There are presently two indications for use of the Esocapsule. The first is for patients with long standing heartburn. The esocapsule looks for changes in the esophagus due to chronic damage. The most common use of the esocapsule is in patients with chronic liver disease. Patients with cirrhosis can develop large blood vessels in the esophagus called varices, which can cause life-threatening bleeding. Patients with cirrhosis should be evaluated for those varices with an esocapsule or upper endoscopy. Medication can be used to help decrease the pressure in varices and decrease the risk of bleeding.

The small bowel is an area of the digestive tract that is located between the stomach and colon (large intestine). There are a few ways to evaluate the small intestine. Like the esophagus test, there is an X-ray test that can evaluate the small bowel with the help of barium. This is known as an upper gastrointestinal series with a small bowel follow through. A more advanced version of this x-ray is called an enteroclysis. Another way to examine the small bowel is with an Enteroscopy. In this procedure, a long endoscope is inserted into the mouth under sedation to examine the small bowel. Instruments can be inserted through the endoscope so that the test is both diagnostic and therapeutic. The small bowel may also be opened up during surgery in order to be examined. This is the most invasive test and is only performed in special circumstances.

The PillCam was developed in order to evaluate the small bowel in a less invasive format. The only preparation is fasting from the night before. The day of the test, a data recorder and eight wires are attached to the patient's lower chest and abdomen. The capsule is then swallowed with water. Most patients do not have difficulty in swallowing the capsule. If there is a problem with swallowing the capsule then the capsule can be inserted with the assistance of an upper endoscopy. After the capsule has been swallowed it moves along the digestive tract in the same way that food moves through the digestive system. The patient can drink water two hours after ingesting the capsule and a light lunch can be eaten about four hours after swallowing the capsule. The total procedure takes about eight hours. You may do your normal activities for the eight hours, other than exercising or doing any heavy lifting during this time. After the eight hours the data recorder and leads are removed, the data recorder is downloaded, and the images are watched in a movie format. There are about 50,000 images. It takes about 60 minutes to read the capsule. The capsule procedure is safe and well tolerated. Capsule endoscopy is avoided in patients with known narrowing of the small intestine and/or history of small bowel obstruction to avoid the capsule becoming stuck and thus causing an intestinal blockage. A small bowel X-ray is sometimes obtained prior to the capsule endoscopy to avoid this complication. Caution must be taken when the patient has a defibrillator or pacemaker.

The PillCam can be used to examine many different conditions of the small bowel. It is most commonly used to evaluate patients with gastrointestinal bleeding. The patient usually has first had an upper endoscopy and a colonoscopy. If no source of bleeding has been identified, the patient may then be referred for a capsule endoscopy. The yield of the capsule endoscopy in these patients is dependent upon the source of the bleeding and how fast it is bleeding. Faster bleeds are more easily identified. The capsule endoscopy can also be used in patients with inflammatory bowel disease or small bowel polyps. Caution is taken when administering the capsule in patients with inflammatory bowel disease because of the increased risk of strictures with Crohn's disease.

66. I've heard that cancer of the esophagus is the fastest rising cancer in the country— is this true, and should I be tested?

There are two general types of cancer of the esophagus—**adenocarcinoma** and **squamous cell carcinoma**. Squamous cell cancer of the esophagus, which is related to smoking, was previously the most common tumor

Adenocarcinoma

A certain type of cancer characterized by the presence of glands when examined under the microscope. This is the kind of cancer associated with Barrett's esophagus.

Squamous cell carcinoma

A type of cancer that can occur in many areas. The commonly seen cancer in the head and neck or esophagus associated with smoking.

141

of the esophagus; this type of esophageal cancer is in decline. Conversely, the incidence of adenocarcinoma of the esophagus has been increasing over the last few decades and now has surpassed that of squamous cell carcinoma. Adenocarcinoma of the esophagus is believed to be due to chronic gastroesophageal reflux of acid.

Adenocarcinoma of the esophagus is believed to be due to chronic gastroesophageal reflux of acid.

Should you be tested? The most common symptom of esophageal cancer is food sticking in the esophagus, otherwise known as dysphagia. In other words, when someone swallows, the food feels like it gets stuck half-way down. However, the vast majority of patients with this difficulty swallowing do not have cancer. The more common causes include benign rings of tissue in the esophagus, acid-related strictures, inflammation of the esophagus (**esophagitis**), or a movement disorder of the esophagus. All patients with dysphagia should have an upper endoscopy. An upper endoscopy is a simple procedure that can be done with minimal sedation. A flexible tube with a camera is inserted into the mouth and then passed into the esophagus, stomach, and first portion of the small intestine (duodenum). If there are any abnormalities that cannot be explained then a biopsy may be performed through a channel in the endoscope. The biopsy is very small (size of the head of pin) and you should not feel it. If there is a narrowing of the esophagus, then the esophagus can be dilated, or stretched. The procedure lasts for about 5 to 10 minutes. Similar to a colonoscopy, you are monitored throughout the procedure and will need a ride home. You should not have anything to eat or drink for at least six hours prior to the procedure.

Esophagitis

Inflammation of the lining of the esophagus that is present in about half of those with chronic reflux symptoms..

There are other non-specific symptoms and signs of esophageal cancer that can warrant investigation, such as gastrointestinal bleeding, a decreased appetite for no obvious reason, or iron deficiency anemia.

Once an esophageal cancer has been detected, further testing needs to be performed to stage the tumor. "Staging" a tumor refers to determining if the tumor is superficial or deep, and whether it has spread beyond the primary organ, which in this case is the esophagus. After an upper endoscopy with biopsies has been performed, the pathologist will evaluate the tissue under a microscope. A CT scan is then performed to determine if the tumor has grown beyond the esophagus. If the CT is negative, meaning that there is no disease outside of the esophagus, then an **endoscopic ultrasound** should be performed. This is similar to the initial endoscopy. It is a slightly larger tube that has a camera and ultrasound probe at the end. The ultrasound allows the doctor to look at the wall of the esophagus and determine how much of the wall of the esophagus is involved. Local lymph nodes are also evaluated at the time of the examination. If the lymph nodes appear suspicious, then a needle can be placed through the wall of the esophagus or stomach to sample the lymph nodes. This will allow a team of doctors (i.e., surgeon, oncologist, radiation oncologist, gastroenterologist) to provide the best treatment. The treatment usually includes a combination of surgery, chemotherapy, and radiation. Patients with very early stage tumors undergo resection as initial treatment. Patients with more advanced tumors should have chemotherapy and radiation first in order to help shrink the tumor. Those patients then will have surgery. This is a major surgery where the esophagus is removed and the stomach is pulled up into the chest. Not all patients are surgical candidates.

Endoscopic ultrasound (EUS)

An instrument similar to endoscopes but also has the capabilities to perform ultrasound. Ultrasound allows investigation of the wall of the lining of the gastrointestinal tract and beyond.

Bernard's comments

I went into Lahey Clinic's Emergency Room. My symptoms were vomiting and diarrhea. both containing blood. After almost 24 hours of observation I was admitted and Dr.

Joyce was called in to do an endoscope on me. Due to all the inflammation, she could not really see what was happening. This was in June. I was scheduled for another endoscope in October. At that time not only did she diagnose that I had "severe dysplasia" Barrett's esophagus but also she discovered a "nodule." After many scopes where she took biopsies and after two re-sections to remove this nodule that did contain cancer, she determined that I would possibly be a candidate for a new treatment called "Barrx." Lahey was not doing this treatment, but by the time I was at a stage that I could have Barrx done, Lahey had gotten their own equipment. Dr. Joyce did the Halo 360 on 9 centimeters of my esophagus that had Barrett's esophagus and she did the Halo 90 on another small area where my esophagus connects to the stomach on a second visit. Because my cancer was detected early and due to all the great care and cooperation I received from Dr. Joyce and the Lahey Clinic staff I was able to "beat" this. My last follow-up endoscope showed a normal, cancer-free, Barrett's free esophagus. Dr. Joyce and all the people I have come in contact with at Lahey Burlington have given me GREAT CARE!! I owe them my life.

67. I've had heartburn for many years—am I at risk of developing esophageal cancer?

Maybe. There is a correlation between heartburn and the risk of esophageal cancer. The number of patients diagnosed with adenocarcinoma is rapidly increasing. It has been associated with acid reflux. The majority of patients with heartburn will not develop esophageal cancer. There are many different definitions of heartburn. Heartburn is typically a burning sensation in the center of the chest that starts at the bottom of the sternum and radiates up the chest. Some patients even experience an acid taste in the mouth. Heartburn is treated with a combination of lifestyle changes and medications. Typical lifestyle changes you can make are small frequent meals, weight loss, avoiding certain foods that promote acid reflux, such as coffee or alcohol, and avoiding lying down immediately after eating. Acid suppressing medications such as antacids, **H2 blockers**, such as ranitidine, and proton pump inhibitors, such as omeprazole, are all used in the management of heartburn.

If you have had heartburn for many years during your lifetime then you should have an upper endoscopy. If you had experienced heartburn several years ago but it now has resolved because you are taking acid suppressing medications, you are still at risk of having chronic damage to your esophagus. You should have an upper endoscopy. At the time of the upper endoscopy, the esophageal lining is carefully examined. The doctor is specifically looking for Barrett's esophagus. Barrett's esophagus is the precursor to esophageal cancer. It is the change in the lining of the esophagus (closest to the stomach) due to repetitive injury from acid reflux. It usually has a distinctive endoscopic appearance but the definite diagnosis is made with sampling the tissue of the affected esophagus.

Barrett's esophagus is most commonly seen in older white males but all patients with frequent heartburn are at risk. Once you have been diagnosed with Barrett's esophagus two things are important: complete heartburn control and follow up endoscopies. For ultimate acid control you should take a proton pump inhibitors once to twice a day for the remainder of your life. The results of the biopsies will determine the interval between endoscopies. The rate of transition of the

H2 blocker

A drug that generally does not require a prescription and is available over the counter. These drugs decrease acid production by the stomach. H2 blockers are effective for esophagitis, GERD, and peptic ulcer disease. They are best used to prevent GERD symptoms and are safe for long-term use. Examples are ranitidine (Zantac), famotidine (Pepcid), nizitadine (Axid), and cimetidine (Tagamet).

cells to cancer is determined by the degree of dysplasia. In patients with no dysplasia, a repeat endoscopy is performed in one year. If there have been no changes then the surveillance endoscopies should be performed every three to five years. If there is low-grade dysplasia, then a repeat endoscopy should be done within a year from the initial examination. If the findings are unchanged, then it is repeated every year. If there is high-grade dysplasia, then a repeat endoscopy is performed within three months.

If you have Barrett's esophagus, it is important that you continue with the acid suppressing medication on a regular basis and have routine upper endoscopies.

If the high-grade dysplasia is confirmed, then you have a few options. Cancer has been detected at the time of surgery for patients with high-grade dysplasia on upper endoscopy. The gold standard would be to an esophagectomy. An esophagectomy is an operation where the esophagus is removed. The second option would be to have an ablative therapy, which is when the Barrett's esophagus is destroyed using various endoscopic techniques. While promising, this is a novel approach in treating dysplasia complicating Barrett's esophagus and should be performed only in centers familiar with its use. If this approach is taken, the patient should continue to have surveillance upper endoscopies every three months. The third option is to do upper endoscopies with biopsies every three months. If a cancer develops, then the patient goes immediately to surgery. The risk of developing cancer in patients with Barrett's esophagus is about 0.4% per year. If the patient is in a surveillance program, then the cancer is usually detected in an earlier stage.

If you have Barrett's esophagus, it is important that you continue with the acid suppressing medication on a regular basis and have routine upper endoscopies.

68. How do you know if you have cancer of the pancreas?

The pancreas is an organ in the abdomen that assists with our digestion of fats and the production of **insulin**. Patients can develop cancer of the pancreas but still have normal function. There are about 30,000 cases of pancreatic cancer each year. It is the fourth leading cause of death. In the majority of cases of pancreatic cancer, the cause is unknown. There are some risk factors associated with pancreatic cancer. Those include older age, tobacco use, some cancer syndromes, and hereditary pancreatitis. Some patients have a family history of pancreatic cancer. If two or more relatives have pancreatic cancer, then there may be increased risk. The majority of patients with pancreatic cancer do not have signs or symptoms until they have advanced disease. The most common presentation of pancreatic cancer is jaundice. Jaundice is characterized by a yellow discoloration of the skin and whites of the eye. The jaundice develops because there is an obstruction of the bile from the liver. The patients usually do not have any abdominal pain. Some pancreatic cancers can present with upper back pain, a decrease in appetite, and weight loss. There has been some association with new onset diabetes or difficult to control blood sugars and pancreatic cancer.

If pancreatic cancer is suspected, then a CT scan is usually the first choice of imaging. A CT scan of the pancreas is an excellent test to identify a mass in the pancreas. Once a mass has been identified, then further characteristics are defined such as size of the tumor, involvement of blood vessels, and enlarged lymph nodes. This information allows the team of doctors to determine the best

Insulin

Hormone produced by specialized cells in the pancreas called islet cells. Insulin has a vital role in the metabolism of sugar-release of insulin into the bloodstream causes blood sugar levels to decrease. Absence of insulin leads to diabetes. Patients with severe chronic pancreatitis can no longer make insulin and therefore become diabetic.

treatment strategy. The mass can also be biopsied. This can be done by a radiologist by passing a needle through the skin (after it has been numbed) into the tumor. More recently, however, a mass in the pancreas is usually biopsied during an endoscopic ultrasound. An endoscopic ultrasound is a specialized type of endoscopy in which the endoscope contains not only a camera to see, but also an ultrasound probe that can be placed right up against the pancreas. Through the endoscopic ultrasound, a needle can be inserted into the tumor for tissue sampling. When patients are jaundiced they may develop itching or infection of the obstructed bile, which is called cholangitis. If any of those two scenarios occur, then an endoscopic retrograde cholangiopancreatography (ERCP) is performed. This again is a specialized type of endoscopy that can relieve the obstruction of bile flow from the liver. In the duodenum the entrance to the bile duct is identified. From here, small instruments are used to get into the bile duct with the assistance of X-ray. Once access is gained to the bile duct, tissue can be obtained from the narrowed (or obstructed) part of the bile duct and a stent can be placed across the stricture. The stent is similar to a plastic straw. The initial stent is usually a temporary stent. This stent will relieve the obstruction thereby relieving the jaundice and itching in one week. The risk of infection is decreased once the obstruction has been relieved. Surgeons prefer not to operate on patients that are still jaundiced so the ERCP may be done before the operation to remove the tumor. The jaundice should be gone prior to starting chemotherapy.

The majority of patients with pancreatic cancer present at an advanced stage. Patients that do have small well-localized tumors are good surgical candidates. The type of surgery involved is dependent on the location of the tumor. Surgery is the best option for cure of the pancreatic cancer. Unfortunately most tumors are not resectable. Those patients who present with larger tumors may require palliative care such as surgery or permanent endoscopic stent placement. Chemotherapy and radiation are not that effective for the treatment of pancreatic cancer. Unfortunately, because pancreatic cancer is usually diagnosed at a late stage, the prognosis of pancreatic cancer is poor.

69. How do you know if you are at risk for developing cancer of the stomach?

Cancer of the stomach is the second most common tumor worldwide. It is commonly seen in Japan. The prevalence of stomach cancer in the United States has been decreasing over the past several decades. There are dietary factors that may increase the risk of developing cancer of the stomach. These include poor nutrition, salted and smoked foods, alcohol, decreased intake of fruits and vegetables, cigarette smoking, and nitrates. Fresh fruits and foods with antioxidants are protective against the development of stomach cancer. There is a bacterium of the stomach called *Helicobacter pylori* that may be associated with stomach cancer. *H. pylori* is the most common chronic bacterial infection in humans. It is thought to be present in about 50% of the world's population. The bacterium is more commonly acquired in developing countries as a child. The majority of patients with *H. pylori* do not have symptoms, nor develop any complications related to *H. pylori*. *H. pylori* can cause ulcers in the stomach. If *H. pylori* is detected it should be eradicated. *H. pylori* is diagnosed with a biopsy of the stomach, blood test, or breath test. The biopsy and breath test are the most accurate for diagnosis, since the blood test remains positive even after treatment. *H. pylori* is treated with a combination of two antibiotics and an acid suppressing medication (such as omeprazole) twice a day for 10 to 14 days. The course of medications should be completed in order to eradicate the bacteria.

Patients with stomach cancer can have a variety of different complaints. The most common symptoms are abdominal pain, weight loss, and nausea. Some patients have a decreased appetite. Others feel full after eating a very small amount of food. There are a few patients that develop bleeding. The patient may vomit blood or pass a dark, tarry bowel movement. When the doctor examines the patient, there may be a mass felt in the abdomen. If cancer of the stomach is suspected, then a combination of an upper endoscopy and CT scan should be performed to confirm the diagnosis. The cancer can be a non-healing ulcer or a mass in the stomach. Biopsies are taken and sent to the pathology laboratory for a diagnosis. In very early stage tumors, the tumor may be removed at the time of endoscopy. In more advanced stage tumors, surgery is a definitive cure for gastric cancer but not all patients are surgical candidates due to the size of the tumor and/or other medical problems. The type of surgery is dependent upon the size and location of the cancer. Chemotherapy and radiation may be helpful for some patients. Unfortunately, stomach cancer often carries a poor prognosis.

70. How do you diagnose cancer of the liver?

The liver is an organ in the right upper part of the abdomen that helps with clearing the blood or toxic substances. The liver produces bile, which helps with the digestion of fats. There are two major types of cancer of liver:

primary and metastatic. **Hepatocellular carcinoma**, also called **hepatoma (HCC)**, is the most common primary cancer of the liver that arises from the cells of the liver. Hepatocellular carcinoma of the liver is most commonly associated with cirrhosis (scarring of the liver). Metastatic cancer to the liver arises when cancerous cells from other areas of the body spread to the liver.

Cirrhosis is the long-term side effect of chronic liver disease. Some of the major causes of the chronic liver disease and cirrhosis include hepatitis B and C, long-term heavy alcohol use, and iron overload. There are also a group of patients who develop scarring of the liver for no clear reason; those patients have cryptogenic cirrhosis. Patients that have cirrhosis of the liver are followed on a routine basis to check for cancer. If a patient with known cirrhosis has worsening symptoms, then hepatocellular carcinoma should be suspected. Hepatocellular carcinoma can present with upper abdominal discomfort and weight loss. The pain may become progressively worse. Other associated symptoms include fatigue, weakness, jaundice or increased abdominal girth related to **ascites** (fluid retention in the abdomen). Hepatocellular carcinoma produces **alpha-fetoprotein (AFP)** which can be detected in the blood. Periodic testing for cancer is performed in patients with cirrhosis given the increased risk of developing cancer. This can be done with a combination of blood tests i.e., alpha-fetoprotein (AFP) and imaging with either ultrasound or MRI. Those tests should be done every three to six months. If cancer is detected in patients with cirrhosis, then the patient may be eligible for a **liver transplantation.**

Another common cause of liver cancer is metastases from other cancers. Metastases are the spread of a tumor from its original site such as digestive tract, lung, or breast to the liver. The symptoms are the same as

Hepatocellular carcinoma

See hepatoma.

Hepatoma (HCC)

Primary cancer of the liver that often occurs in the setting of cirrhosis.

Ascites

Abnormal fluid accumulation in the abdomen that can develop when the liver does not function properly.

Alpha-fetoprotein (AFP)

A blood test that is often elevated in patients who have liver cancer.

Liver transplant

A major surgical procedure that involves the removal of a diseased liver and the insertion of a healthy liver.

with primary liver cancer. Liver metastases are usually detected through dedicated X-rays, such as ultrasound, CT scan, or MRI. If there is a suspected lesion in the liver, then a biopsy is usually performed. This biopsy is performed through the skin under X-ray guidance. The biopsy can usually identify the origin of the tumor.

There are a variety of different treatments for hepatocellular carcinoma. Patients with cirrhosis may be candidates for a liver transplantation. The eligibility for a liver transplantation is dependent upon the severity of the liver disease and the size and location of the tumor(s) in the liver. Patients without underlying liver disease may also be candidates for surgical resection. Again the surgery is dependent upon the size and location of the tumor(s). If surgery is not an option there are other less invasive methods that may be helpful. Ablative therapy can be done to help shrink the tumor. Another method is to cut off the blood supply to the tumor. Injecting chemotherapy into the lesion can also help to shrink the lesion. Those latter methods are palliative in that they help control the tumor but are not curative.

The eligibility for a liver transplantation is dependent upon the severity of the liver disease and the size and location of the tumor(s) in the liver.

71. Can you do anything to prevent cancer of the digestive system?

Gastrointestinal cancers account for about one third of all cancers diagnosed. Unfortunately, there are no definitive ways to prevent the development or cancer of the gastrointestinal tract, liver, or pancreas. There are some who believe that dietary supplements may reduce the likelihood of developing cancer. And while the evidence for dietary supplements in preventing of treating cancer is limited, overall a healthy diet and exercise are the keys for improved general health.

Selenium

Selenium is a trace mineral. Selenium is available in seafood, meat, and plant foods. The association between the protective effects of selenium was first recognized in the 1960s. There are small studies that show that selenium may decrease the risk of esophageal carcinoma and colon cancer. In animal studies, the results are not that promising but there may be some benefit with human trials. The daily recommended dose of selenium in the average person is 70 micrograms. Most people are able to ingest about 100 micrograms in their diet. The dose recommended in the studies for cancer prevention is 200 micrograms of selenium once a day. Selenium may also be protective against prostate and lung cancer.

Antioxidant Vitamins

There are a variety of different agents that have antioxidant effects. Antioxidant vitamins include vitamins A, C, and E. Antioxidants are found in a diet rich in fruits and vegetables. Antioxidants affect the body's method of dealing with toxic free radicals (or unstable cells) that may play a role in the development of cancer. Free radicals have been associated with cigarette smoking, pollution, sun exposure, and food digestion. There are varying reports as to the effectiveness of antioxidants and the prevention of cancer. More clinical trials are needed before recommendations can be made to take additional antioxidants beyond the standard intake. At this time, a diet rich in fruits and vegetables is recommended for everyone. Some foods that are particularly high in antioxidants include yellow and orange foods, green leafy vegetables, and certain fruits such as strawberries, kiwi fruit, and plums. Tomatoes are a good source of lycopene, which is also an antioxidant.

Folate

Folate is a vitamin that is found in green leafy vegetables, fruits, cereals, grains, nuts, and meats. It is commonly recommended in pregnant females as part of the prenatal vitamins to prevent neural tube defects. Folate may help to prevent damage of DNA, which may then help to prevent cancer. In both the Health Professionals Study and the Nurses' Health Study, folate has been shown to potentially decrease the risk of colon cancer. The results were more significant in men that drink alcohol (Author's note: Alcohol should always be used in moderation).

Calcium

Calcium may control the changes in cells in order to prevent cancer. Calcium has been studied in the higher risk groups of patients with colon cancer. Those patients include familial polyp syndromes or patients with a personal history of colonic polyps. The standard dose that was used in the studies was from 1200 to 1500 mg of elemental calcium. Again, the results are mixed as to the effectiveness of calcium. The results have been promising in the preclinical setting. There are ongoing studies in regards to calcium and the effect on colorectal cancer.

NSAIDs

Anti-inflammatory medications such as aspirin or suldinac have been shown to decrease the risk of cancer. It is thought to be related to the cyclooxygenase inhibition through the COX-2 enzyme. Specific COX-2 inhibitors such as Celebrex were recommended in some high-risk patients. Unfortunately, some of the COX-2 inhibitors have been associated with increased cardiovascular events. Multiple studies have shown that the regular use of NSAIDs may help to decrease the risk of esophageal and colon cancer. The benefits are seen in patients that take the medicine for greater than 10 years and at higher doses. Unfortunately, there are some risks associated with the use of NSAIDs such as gastrointestinal bleeding or hemorrhagic strokes. NSAIDs are not routinely recommended in the average risk patients but may be helpful in higher risk patients.

Overall it is difficult to recommend any one of these agents that have a definite preventative effect. It is important to eating a healthy diet with fruits and vegetables and to avoid certain carcinogens, such as tobacco and alcohol.

PART SEVEN

The Pancreas and Gallbladder

Stephen J. Heller, MD

What is acute pancreatitis?

What are gallstones?

My doctor says that I need to have an ERCP to remove a gallstone from the bile duct—what is an ERCP?

More . . .

72. What is the pancreas and what does it do?

The pancreas is an oblong organ that sits in the upper abdomen. It is typically between 6 and 10 inches long, and is located immediately behind the stomach and next to the duodenum (small intestine). It is divided into three parts: the head, body and tail.

The functions of the pancreas can be divided into two main categories. Specialized cells in the pancreas called **islet cells** control the level of blood sugar. These cells produce hormones called insulin and **glucagon**. These substances are released directly into the bloodstream. The other cells in the pancreas produce enzymes that aid in digestion of food: **amylase**, **lipase**, **trypsin** and **chymotrypsin**. These enzymes are released into the main duct of the pancreas. This duct drains directly into the small intestine, where digestion takes place.

It is possible to live without a pancreas. Insulin injections are required to control the diabetes that always occurs. Pancreas enzymes for digestion can be taken in pill form to substitute for the body's production of these enzymes. In severe cases of chronic pancreatitis, with marked destruction of the pancreas, patients may develop diabetes as well as weight loss and malnutrition related to impaired digestion of nutrients.

73. What is acute pancreatitis?

Acute pancreatitis is an inflammatory condition of the pancreas. Patients generally develop severe abdominal pain fairly suddenly. The pain is most often located in the center of the upper abdomen, between the navel and the lower end of the breastbone. Sometimes the pain will be in the upper abdomen but on the left or right side. The pain can also occur lower in the abdomen, at about the level of the navel.

The pain often bores through from the front of the abdomen to the back. In many cases, the pain is accompanied by nausea and vomiting. There may be fevers too, and patients generally see a doctor within a day or so of the beginning of the pain. Often the severity of the pain prompts a visit to the emergency room.

Most cases of acute pancreatitis require admission to the hospital. However, the majority of time, even though the initial symptoms are quite severe, the situation improves quickly and patients stay in the hospital for only a few days. Less commonly, the pain persists, requiring a longer stay in the hospital.

Most cases of acute pancreatitis require admission to the hospital.

About one in ten cases of acute pancreatitis is more serious. The inflammation of the pancreas will lead to impairment in lung or kidney function or infection. These issues may in turn require transfer to an intensive care unit. Sometimes a breathing tube or kidney dialysis is needed. Severe cases of acute pancreatitis can be life-threatening.

Severe acute pancreatitis may lead to death of pancreatic tissue. This dead tissue can become infected, which is potentially fatal. This type of infection may not be treatable with antibiotics alone, but instead requires surgery to remove the infected tissue. Large collections of fluid called **pseudocysts** can also develop when pancreatitis is severe. These collections of fluid can become infected or block the passage of food through the digestive tract. Pseudocysts often resolve on their own over the course of weeks to months, but when a pseudocyst

Pseudocysts
Fluid-filled collection of tissue in or adjacent to the pancreas.

159

fails to resolve, drainage is required. Drainage can be accomplished either with surgery or less invasive means such as endoscopy performed by a gastroenterologist, or drainage through the skin performed by a radiologist.

74. How is acute pancreatitis diagnosed?

Acute pancreatitis is suspected by the physician when a patient describes the sudden development of severe pain in the upper abdomen. Because pancreatitis is usually caused by either alcohol or gallstones, the suspicion for acute pancreatitis is increased when the patient has ingested a large amount of alcohol, or when the patient is known to have gallstones.

The physical examination is important in diagnosing acute pancreatitis. Patients generally appear uncomfortable from the pain and nausea. There may be a rapid heart rate or elevated blood pressure from the pain, nausea and vomiting, and dehydration. There may also be a fever, although this is typically mild. Examination of the upper abdomen reveals tenderness which may be severe.

Because the pancreas releases its enzymes into the bloodstream during acute pancreatitis, detection of elevation in these enzymes is crucial for the diagnosis of acute pancreatitis. The most common blood test is the amylase, and sometimes the lipase is checked too. These are enzymes produced by the pancreas that spill into the bloodstream during acute pancreatitis. It is normal to have some amylase or lipase in the bloodstream; however, the levels of at least one of these enzymes should be at least 3 times the maximum normal level in order to clinch the diagnosis of acute pancreatitis. The amylase and lipase tests each have advantages and disadvantages. The amylase is elevated earlier in the illness which is more useful since patients come to the doctor soon after the pain begins. However, elevation in amylase is not unique to acute pancreatitis (i.e., amylase may be elevated in other gastrointestinal disorders such as gallbladder infection). Furthermore, amylase is also normally found in saliva, and disorders of the salivary glands can also raise the level of amylase in the blood and confuse the issue. Lipase is more specific to the pancreas, but the level of lipase may rise later in the illness and thus is not always as helpful in the early setting.

Radiologic imaging of the abdomen is also very important in diagnosing acute pancreatitis. What particular test is ordered by the physician may depend on the hospital. Ultrasound, CAT scan and MRI are all capable of diagnosing acute pancreatitis. These tests can each identify the hallmarks of acute pancreatitis, which are swelling or enlargement of the pancreas and abnormal fluid around the pancreas. Each test has advantages and disadvantages—you can discuss this with your doctor.

75. What causes acute pancreatitis?

Alcohol and gallstones are by far the most common causes of acute pancreatitis. More than 80% of cases of acute pancreatitis in the United States are caused by either alcohol or gallstones. Alcohol has a damaging effect on the pancreas. The amount of ingested alcohol necessary to cause acute pancreatitis is generally large. Most patients who have acute pancreatitis related to alcohol drink considerable amounts of alcohol on a chronic basis. The attack of acute pancreatitis occurs within a few days of alcohol ingestion.

Alcohol has a damaging effect on the pancreas.

Gallstones are a frequent cause of acute pancreatitis. This occurs when a gallstone from gallbladder escapes from the gallbladder into the bile duct. The bile duct joins with the duct from the pancreas just before both ducts empty into the small intestine. When a gallstone blocks the pancreatic duct, pancreatitis can result. Because the bile duct and the pancreatic duct are small, it is usually small gallstones that cause acute pancreatitis.

There are many less common causes of acute pancreatitis: elevated blood levels of triglycerides or calcium, certain medications, congenital abnormalities of the pancreas, physical injury to the pancreas, and rare infections. Pancreatitis may occur as a complication of surgery, particularly surgery involving structures neighboring the pancreas such as the kidneys. Pancreatitis may follow a type of endoscopy looking at the pancreas called an ERCP. This is ironic because ERCP is commonly performed to evaluate the pancreas in the hopes of treating disorders of the pancreas or bile duct, but the procedure itself causes acute pancreatitis in about one in twenty cases. Tumors of the pancreas can cause acute pancreatitis. In rare circumstances, the first sign of a tumor of the pancreas will be an attack of acute pancreatitis.

76. How is acute pancreatitis treated?

Patients are usually admitted to the hospital for treatment of acute pancreatitis. Treatment of acute pancreatitis is supportive. A principle of treatment is resting the pancreas; because the pancreas is stimulated by eating, patients are treated with "nothing by mouth" or NPO initially. In order to maintain adequate hydration, intravenous fluids are given. Dehydration may be compounded by loss of fluids from vomiting. The pain from acute pancreatitis can be intense. Narcotics such as morphine, meperidine (Demerol) or dilaudid are given intravenously. Medication for nausea is also given. These medications are effective in controlling these symptoms. If vomiting is persistent, a plastic tube may be placed from the nose to the stomach to remove fluid from the stomach (an "NG tube"). Unfortunately, at the present time there is no specific treatment that physicians can use that directly targets the inflammation of the pancreas. However, with the supportive treatment outlined above, patients usually get better in a few days and are discharged from the hospital.

In a minority of cases, acute pancreatitis can become severe. Blood pressure can become dangerously low. There can be impairment of lung and kidney function and serious infection may develop. In these cases, careful monitoring in the intensive care unit is mandatory. If the impairment in lung function is severe enough, placement of a breathing tube may be necessary. In some cases, dialysis is needed due to kidney failure. In severe cases of acute pancreatitis, some or all of the pancreatic tissue dies. This dead pancreatic tissue is at high risk for become infected. When infection of this tissue occurs, treatment with antibiotics alone is not sufficient and surgery is necessary. Fluid-filled collections of tissue called pseudocysts may form. These can also become infected, or they can block the flow of nutrients through the digestive tract. These pseudocysts can be treated either with surgery or with a special type of drainage procedure performed either with an endoscopy whereby the pseudocyst is drained through the stomach, or a specialized radiologist will place a drain in the pseudocyst under CAT scan guidance.

There is a role for a specialized type of endoscopy called ERCP in some cases of acute pancreatitis related to gallstones. When the physician believes that the gallstone is stuck in the bile duct where it joins the pancreatic duct, he or she may recommend an endoscopy called ERCP (endoscopic retrograde cholangiopancreatography) to prevent infection from forming in the bile duct. Performing this specialized procedure, the physician advances a flexible endoscope into the small intestine at the point where the bile duct and pancreatic duct join and drain into the small intestine. A catheter is threaded into the opening of these ducts and the opening is enlarged using a technique called sphincterotomy. The stone is pulled out and allowed to pass through the intestine.

77. What is chronic pancreatitis?

Chronic pancreatitis is a chronic inflammatory condition which results in destruction to the pancreatic tissue. Depending on the severity of the case varying amounts of the pancreas are destroyed. This condition is often very painful, debilitating and difficult to treat.

By far the most common cause of chronic pancreatitis is alcohol abuse. In most cases, patients with chronic pancreatitis from alcohol have drunk large amounts of alcohol for many years. Other rarer causes of chronic pancreatitis include hypertriglyceridemia, tropical pancreatitis which is found only in a few specific locations, such as India. There is a rare, hereditary form of chronic pancreatitis. The genes responsible for this disorder have been identified. In contrast to chronic pancreatitis, which generally afflicts individuals in early adulthood and middle age, hereditary pancreatitis strikes earlier in life. Much attention has also been given to cystic fibrosis as a cause of chronic pancreatitis. Individuals who do not have the full-blown disease of cystic fibrosis, but carry one of the two genes necessary for the disease (called heterozygotes) may have chronic pancreatitis but no other signs of cystic fibrosis.

The type of damage to the pancreas that occurs in chronic pancreatitis is variable. Sometimes the inflammation is on a microscopic level and difficult to see with radiologic tests such as CAT scans. In other cases, the pancreas is obviously inflamed and destroyed. The main pancreatic duct is often abnormally enlarged or alternatively may be have narrowed areas called strictures. There may be calcium deposits in the pancreas tissue which can be seen even with a standard X-ray of the abdomen. Sometimes plugs of thick material can accumulate in the pancreatic duct and block the outflow of pancreatic juice, thereby contributing to the pain.

78. How is chronic pancreatitis diagnosed?

The physician suspects chronic pancreatitis in the setting of chronic severe pain in the upper abdomen, particularly in patients with a history of excessive alcohol intake. However, not all patients with chronic pancreatitis have a history of alcohol abuse. As in acute pancreatitis, the pain will often radiate to the back and can be triggered by eating. Other signs and symptoms to suggest chronic pancreatitis include weight loss and evidence of oily, foul-smelling stools (called **steatorrhea**), which result from loss of pancreatic digestive enzymes.

...not all patients with chronic pancreatitis have a history of alcohol abuse.

Steatorrhea
Loose, oily stools containing fat.

Unlike acute pancreatitis, in which the amylase and/or lipase are elevated, in chronic pancreatitis the amylase and lipase blood levels are usually normal. In severe chronic pancreatitis, impairment of digestion is confirmed by collection of stool for 3 days and measuring the fat content. Obviously this test is inconvenient to perform (to say the least) and the results may be normal in mild or moderate cases. Tests to check pancreas enzyme levels in the stool are also limited in that they tend to be elevated only in severe cases of chronic pancreatitis, when the diagnosis was never in doubt in the first place.

Secretin test

A test to measure how well the pancreas is functioning.

Nasograstic tube

A long, flexible tube that passes through the nose into the stomach.

Many clinicians consider the "gold standard" test for chronic pancreatitis to be the **secretin test**. This examination is invasive (a **nasogastric tube** is placed into the small intestine), cumbersome and time-consuming. It is performed at only a few centers and is therefore not a practical option for most patients.

The diagnosis of chronic pancreatitis is generally confirmed by some type of imaging test to visualize the pancreas. A routine X-ray of the abdomen may demonstrate calcium deposits in the pancreas, a sign of chronic pancreatitis. More commonly, CT scan or MRI is necessary to confirm the diagnosis. The findings of chronic pancreatitis are variable. These imaging tests may show inflammation or atrophy of the pancreas. The main duct draining the pancreatic juice (called the pancreatic duct) may be widened, or may demonstrate focal areas of narrowing or stones within the duct. MRI is particularly useful for evaluating the pancreatic duct.

ERCP can also be used as a diagnostic test to identify the abnormalities of the pancreatic duct seen in chronic pancreatitis. However, MRI provides nearly the same information without the risk of an invasive procedure, so it has largely replaced ERCP as the best diagnostic test for evaluating the pancreatic duct.

79. How is chronic pancreatitis treated?

The treatment of chronic pancreatitis is challenging. The goals of treatment are improvement in pain and treatment of weight loss and malnutrition. The pain from chronic pancreatitis is usually severe enough to require strong pain-killing medication, frequently narcotics. Initially over-the-counter analgesics are tried but are generally ineffective. Medications such as darvocet, codeine and Vicodin are used with some success. In severe cases, strong narcotics such as oxycodone, Demerol, and morphine are necessary to control the pain. In patients with intermittent pain, the physician prescribes medication to take on an as-needed basis only when the pain occurs. In patients with chronic pain, the physician prescribes long-acting narcotics to take on a daily basis, in the hope of making the pain manageable or preventing pain before it starts.

Pancreatic enzymes are prescribed and are effective in treating the impaired digestion that occurs in severe chronic pancreatitis. These enzymes come in a variety of brand names and preparations. Often a medication to suppress acid production from the stomach is prescribed in conjunction with the enzymes, in order to prevent stomach acid from breaking down the enzymes in the stomach. The role of pancreas enzymes in treating the pain from chronic pancreatitis is controversial. Some physicians believe that pancreas enzymes are helpful in treating the pain from chronic pancreatitis because when the enzymes are given the pancreas "rests" and the pancreas in the resting state is less likely to be irritated and trigger pain. Because pancreatic enzymes have few side effects, clinicians often give them a try in treating the pain in chronic pancreatitis, but often without success.

When more than 90% of the pancreas is destroyed, diabetes results. In these cases, insulin injections are required to control blood sugar.

In selected cases there is a role for endoscopic or surgical treatment of chronic pancreatitis. In some cases of chronic pancreatitis, stones form in the pancreatic duct and can block the flow of pancreatic juice into the small intestine. This blockage can contribute to the pain in this condition. A specific type of endoscopy called an ERCP (see below) can be used to remove the stones from the main pancreatic duct. Sometimes a technique called **extracorporeal shock-wave lithotripsy (ESWL)** is used first to fragment the stones into smaller pieces so that they can be more easily removed by ERCP. This technique is often performed by urologists because it is most commonly used in the treatment of kidney stones.

Extracorporeal shock wave lithotripsy (ESWL)

Noninvasive technique using high-energy sound waves to break up gallstones.

If initial measures such as medication and avoiding alcohol are unsuccessful, and symptoms are disabling, surgery may be considered for chronic pancreatitis. Surgery is not a suitable option for chronic pancreatitis in all cases. There are different operations that the surgeon will consider. Surgery on the pancreas can be complex and carry significant risk. It is recommended that patients choose a surgeon who specializes in diseases of the pancreas and has experience in pancreatic surgery.

80. How are gallstones diagnosed?

Gallstones are most commonly diagnosed by a form of X-ray examination. The most common tests that detect gallstones are ultrasound, CAT scan and MRI. Of these examinations, ultrasound is the simplest to perform. The radiologist (or technician) places an ultrasound probe over the right side of the upper abdomen and images are taken. In addition to the gallbladder, an ultrasound provides a good look at the liver and kidneys. Sometimes the pancreas is seen on ultrasound; however, because ultrasound waves do not travel through gas, and the gas-filled bowel often lies directly above the pancreas, often times the pancreas is not well seen on ultrasound.

Gallstones can also be seen on a CAT scan of the abdomen. Having a CAT scan usually requires the patient to drink a white liquid which is an X-ray contrast agent. This outlines the intestine and helps the radiologist distinguish the intestine from other organs in the abdomen. In most cases contrast is given intravenously as well, which helps better define the abdominal organs. An advantage of CAT scan over ultrasound is that CAT scan visualizes all the abdominal organs. For example, the pancreas is not often well seen on ultrasound but is very well seen on CAT scan. A disadvantage of CAT scan compared with ultrasound is that undergoing CAT scan requires drinking the contrast agent and generally receiving the intravenous contrast agent. Receiving intravenous contrast carries a small risk of an allergic reaction, which in rare cases can be serious.

Magnetic resonance imaging or MRI can also be used to diagnose gallstones. MRI, like CAT scan, provides accurate images of the entire abdomen. MRI offers a specific advantage over CAT scan: it can provide special pictures called an MRCP (magnetic resonance cholangiopancreatography). These images provide excellent pictures not only of the gallbladder but also of the common bile duct. Gallstones may sit in the bile duct as well as the gallbladder. MRI offers the unique ability to identify gallstones in both the bile duct and gallbladder much more accurately than either CAT scan or ultrasound. One potential drawback of MRI is that patients who have pacemakers or who have undergone certain types of brain surgery may not be eligible for this type of examination. In addition, undergoing MRI requires staying motionless in a narrow tube for up to 45 minutes. For patients who are claustrophobic this can be very anxiety-provoking, if not impossible. Sometimes the physician will prescribe a mild tranquilizer in these patients to make the procedure more tolerable.

Ultrasound, CAT scan and MRI are all reasonably good in diagnosing gallstones in the gallbladder. It might be surprising to learn that ultrasound, although the least "high-tech" of these three techniques, is actually the best at diagnosing gallstones in the gallbladder. If the doctor is most interested in looking for gallstones in the gallbladder, ultrasound is an excellent test. MRI is the best test for diagnosing gallstones in the bile duct.

81. What is the gallbladder?

The gallbladder is a green, pear-shaped organ that sits next to the liver in the right upper abdomen. It is about 3 to 5 inches long in humans. The function of the gallbladder is to store bile which is produced by the liver. The gallbladder contracts and releases bile into the intestine after meals. Bile has an important role in digesting fats. Despite these important-sounding functions, humans can live normal, healthy lives after the gallbladder has been removed surgically. The functions of the gallbladder are assumed by the liver and bile ducts after the gallbladder has been removed.

82. What are gallstones?

Gallstones range in size from tiny particles like grains of sand up to firm concretions 2 inches in diameter. Sometimes a jelly-like material forms which is called gallbladder sludge. Although sludge is liquid and stones are solid, sludge can cause the very same problems as stones. Most gallstones are cholesterol stones, which are composed primarily of cholesterol. A minority of stones are pigment stones, which are made up of multiple components of bile including calcium and bilirubin. These substances naturally occur in bile.

Gallstones form when there is an imbalance in the components of bile. This results in solid material precipitating out of the bile to form stones.

Who is at risk for developing stones? The risk factors for cholesterol and pigment stones are different. Women are two to three times as likely as men to develop cholesterol stones. Pregnancy is a risk factor for gallstones. Certain ethnic groups such as Native Americans have a higher rate of gallstones. African-Americans are less likely than whites to develop gallstones. Obesity but also rapid weight loss have been associated with gallstone formation. Because gallstones rarely disappear on their own, gallstones are more commonly seen in older people. Several drugs, most notably female hormones, increase the risk of gallstone formation.

Women are two to three times as likely as men to develop cholesterol stones.

The risk factors for pigment stones are different from cholesterol stones. Pigment stones account for no more than 25% of stones in the United States but they account for a much higher percentage of gallstones among Asian-Americans. Risk factors for pigment stones include blood disorders in which red blood cells are destroyed, releasing bilirubin which creates an imbalance in the composition of bile leading to stone precipitation. Cirrhosis of the liver can also lead to pigment stones. Some individuals have chronic infection of the bile ducts, which is known to cause pigment stones. This condition is much more common in Asia than the United States.

Although the cholesterol and pigment stones are different in terms of how they are formed, once they are formed they cause very similar problems.

83. My doctor found gallstones on an ultrasound test but I don't have any abdominal pain. Should I be concerned?

Gallstones are often found in people without any symptoms.

Gallstones are often found in people without any symptoms. For example, patients having a radiologic examination of the abdomen for another reason may be given the diagnosis of "incidental" gallstones. Most individuals with gallstones diagnosed in this manner will never develop symptoms. However, in a minority of individuals, symptoms will occur over time. Studies have shown that in people with gallstones but no symptoms, about one in five will develop a problem from the gallstones over one's lifetime. Physicians sometimes tell patients that out of one hundred people with asymptomatic gallstones, each year between two and five will develop symptoms. In most patients, the first sign of a problem from gallstones is abdominal pain without any serious complications. Once this occurs, the gallbladder is generally removed without difficulty and the patient's symptoms subside.

84. How are gallstones treated?

The best treatment for gallstones in the gallbladder is surgery. Once the gallbladder is removed, most patients have no further problems from gallstones. The risk of problems following gallbladder removal does not decline to zero, however, because stones can form in the bile duct. Unlike the gallbladder, the bile duct is essential for survival and cannot be removed.

The traditional operation for removing the gallbladder involves making an incision in the right upper abdomen. This operation is tried and true but requires several days in the hospital and about one month before returning to work.

This surgery, often called "open" **cholecystectomy** (removal of the gallbladder) has been replaced by laparoscopic cholecystectomy as the "gold standard" for the treatment of gallstones. In this operation, the surgeon removes the gall bladder without a large incision. Instead, four much smaller incisions are made and the gallbladder is removed with the use of a video camera and other specialized instruments. The laparoscopic approach is still surgery and requires general anesthesia. However, because of the much smaller incisions, patients usually can either go home the same day of the operation or sometimes stay one night in the hospital. Patients typically return to work in one to two weeks.

Cholecystectomy
Surgical removal of the gallbladder.

The obvious advantages of the laparoscopic approach to removing the gallbladder make this the first choice for both patients and physicians. But in some cases the laparoscopic approach is not impossible and the surgeon has no choice but to open the abdomen and perform the traditional operation. For example, a large amount of scar tissue in the abdomen can obstruct the surgeon's ability to dissect the gallbladder out safely using the laparoscopic technique.

Surgery is the preferred option for the vast majority of patients with problems related to gallstones. A problem arises when a patient is felt to be too high a risk to undergo an operation. Or occasionally a patient is dead-set against having surgery. There are a few other options available. In a patient with an infected gallbladder (acute cholecystitis), who is believed to be at high risk for surgery, the radiologist may place a tube through the skin into the gallbladder called a percutaneous **cholecystostomy**. This tube will drain the infection and together with antibiotics can provide temporary treatment.

Cholecystostomy

Drainage tube placed from the skin directly into the gallbladder.

Another option is medical therapy in the form of pills to dissolve stones. This treatment was more popular before the advent of laparoscopic surgery. The most commonly used medication is ursodeoxycholic acid. This medication changes the composition of bile and can dissolve gallstones. Unfortunately, only a fraction of patients with gallstones are even candidates for this form of treatment. Patients must take medication for up to 2 years and even then the medication is successful only about half the time. And over several years after stopping treatment, stones will re-form in 50% of individuals.

A technique called extracorporeal shock-wave lithotripsy (ESWL) has been used as an alternative to surgery. In this technique, shock waves are applied to the gallstones and fragment or break them into small pieces. Then, medical therapy such as ursodeoxycholic acid is prescribed. This treatment, like medical therapy alone, is limited by the high rate of recurrent problems after the treatment is discontinued. Surgery is the treatment of choice in the patient who can tolerate it.

85. What is an ERCP?

ERCP is an abbreviation for endoscopic retrograde cholangiopancreatography. ERCP is an endoscopy procedure with the objective of examining the bile duct or pancreatic duct.

The most common reason for performing an ERCP is when the physician suspects a stone in the bile duct. When patients have pain in the upper abdomen, in conjunction with enlargement of the bile duct on imaging such as ultrasound or CT scan, elevation in liver function tests on blood work, or jaundice, a bile duct stone is a strong possibility. ERCP is also performed when there is suspicion for a blockage in the bile duct, either from benign inflammation or a tumor.

The pancreatic duct can also be examined by ERCP, most commonly in patients with chronic pancreatitis with stones in the pancreatic duct. ERCP may be useful in removing such stones, which can be useful in treating the pain from chronic pancreatitis in selected patients.

ERCP is generally performed as an outpatient, unless the patient is already admitted to the hospital. The procedure is performed with an anesthetic, either "conscious sedation" given through an intravenous catheter, or general anesthesia administered by an anesthesiologist. Local anesthetic spray is applied to the throat to numb the gag reflex. The test generally takes between thirty and ninety minutes. Once the patient is comfortably sedated, a flexible endoscope is advanced into the mouth, through the esophagus and stomach, and into the small intestine. The opening into the bile duct and pancreatic duct (called the **ampulla of Vater**) is identified in the small intestine. The physician then passes a thin catheter under direct X-ray guidance directly into

The most common reason for performing an ERCP is when the physician suspects a stone in the bile duct.

Ampulla of Vater

Opening of the small intestine where the bile duct and pancreatic duct join and drain into the small intestine.

the desired duct. Dye is injected into the duct and X-ray images are taken. If a stone is identified, it is removed by enlarging the opening to the bile duct (called a sphincterotomy) and pulling the stone out of the duct. The stone is left in the intestine where it should pass without difficulty. If a blockage is identified, a tissue sample may be obtained and sent for analysis. A plastic or expandable metal tube called a stent may also be left in the bile duct to allow bile to drain from the liver and bypass the obstruction.

ERCP is more invasive than a routine endoscopic procedure and carries a higher risk of complications. The most frequent complication is acute pancreatitis, which occurs after about 5–10% of cases. In most cases, pancreatitis following ERCP requires admission to the hospital for a few days. Rarely, the illness can be severe or even life-threatening. Bleeding, infection and perforation of the intestine can also occur but are less common. Rarely, blood transfusions or surgery are necessary to manage these complications. ERCP is an advanced endoscopic procedure that is best performed by a physician experienced in this examination.

PART EIGHT

The Liver

Stephen C. Fabry, MD

How common is liver disease?

What is a liver biopsy?

Can prescribed or over-the-counter drugs
affect the liver?

More . . .

86. What is the liver and what does it do?

The liver is an amazing and vital organ. The largest organ in the body, it is located on the right side of the abdomen underneath the rib cage. The average person's liver weighs between three and five pounds. The liver has a complicated blood supply, receiving blood from the **hepatic** artery and the portal vein. The hepatic artery brings oxygen-rich blood from the heart. The portal vein drains blood from the digestive system into the liver. The hepatic vein carries blood from the liver back to the heart. The bile duct carries bile from the liver into the small intestine.

Everyone is born with only one liver, so it is important to keep it functioning well. The liver performs many essential functions that are necessary for life. These functions include removing poisons and drugs from the body, manufacturing many different types of proteins, storing energy, fighting infections, storing iron reserves, storing minerals and vitamins, and producing bile to help digest food.

The liver processes almost all foods, drugs, and toxins that enter the body into either safer or more usable substances. It produces many proteins, including clotting factors, **albumin** (which accounts for most of the protein in blood), and a variety of proteins that are used as transporters and receptors throughout the body. The liver serves as a major site of energy storage that can be tapped by other parts of the body when necessary. Glucose is the main source of energy for human cells. The liver converts excess glucose to glycogen for storage. Glycogen is then converted back to glucose when energy is needed. In addition to storing glycogen, the liver also stores many other substances including iron, copper, and

Hepatic

A term used to refer to anything pertaining to the liver.

Everyone is born with only one liver, so it is important to keep it functioning well.

Albumin

A protein produced by the liver that accounts for most of the protein in blood.

vitamin B12. The liver produces and excretes bile into the intestines. Bile is necessary for proper absorption of fats including the fat-soluble vitamins A, D, E, and K.

87. How common is liver disease?

Liver disease is very common in the United States. Approximately 25,000,000 Americans have a liver related disorder and about 27,000 Americans die each year from chronic liver diseases. The Centers for Disease Control (CDC) estimates that there were 513,000 hospital discharges for chronic liver disease or cirrhosis in 2004. The CDC lists chronic liver disease and cirrhosis as the seventh leading cause of death in the 25–44 years and the 45–64 years age groups. The most common liver diseases in the United States include nonalcoholic steatohepatitis (fatty liver), hepatitis A, hepatitis B, hepatitis C, iron overload, and immune liver disorders.

Fatty liver is by far the most common liver disease in our country. In one large study, over 2,000 patients underwent proton (H1)-nuclear magnetic resonance (NMR) spectroscopy (a fancy X-ray of the liver) and 31% were found to have fatty liver. Most (79%) of the patients had normal liver blood tests. In another large study, over 15,000 adults had blood tests and 5.5% were found to have elevated liver enzymes presumably from fatty liver. There were an estimated 42,000 new cases of hepatitis A in 2005 but luckily hepatitis A never becomes a chronic problem and almost all patients recover completely. Widespread vaccination against hepatitis A has significantly decreased the number of new infections. Chronic hepatitis B is a major worldwide health problem. There are an estimated 350 million people worldwide with chronic hepatitis B. In the United States, there are an estimated 1.25 million people with chronic infection. Hepatitis C is more common in the United States with an estimated 3.9 million people infected. The World Health Organization estimates that there are 170 million people worldwide with chronic hepatitis C. Iron overload (or hemochromatosis) is more common in certain areas of the world. Caucasians of Northern European descent are most likely to be affected. Hemochromatosis is a genetic condition in which the affected individual receives an abnormal gene from both parents. In the United States about 0.5% of the population (1 out of 200) carry two copies of the hemochromatosis gene and are at risk for developing clinical disease. Immune liver diseases include autoimmune hepatitis, primary biliary cirrhosis, and **primary sclerosing cholangitis (PSC)** and are very rare.

Primary sclerosing cholangitis (PSC)

Inflammation and scarring of the bile ducts within the liver; can be seen in IBD.

88. How do you know if you have liver disease?

Liver disease can be diagnosed through a variety of different situations. The first major distinction is whether a patient has a new and sudden development of a liver disease or a chronic liver disease. New liver disease (usually called acute hepatitis) is less common and usually fairly obvious. Patients with no previous history of liver problems develop jaundice, dark urine, light stools, loss of appetite, and general fatigue. Most patients recover completely although some patients will transition into a chronic hepatitis and a very few patients (about 2,000 a year in the United States) will develop liver failure and need a liver transplant. The most common causes of acute hepatitis are viruses such as hepatitis A and hepatitis B, medications such as acetaminophen (found in Tylenol and other over the counter medications), and decreased blood flow to the liver.

Most patients who are diagnosed with liver disease have a chronic problem that may have been present for many years. Patients can be diagnosed with liver disease either before or after symptoms have developed. Most patients do not develop symptoms from liver disease until cirrhosis has developed. Patients with no symptoms are diagnosed either incidentally or because of screening. Many people will have blood tests or X-rays done for other reasons and are found to incidentally have abnormalities that lead to the diagnosis of a chronic liver disease. Some people are diagnosed with liver disease when their doctor takes a history and finds a risk factor such as a family history of liver problems. Patients with symptoms are obviously diagnosed when they present to their doctor because of a specific complaint. Symptoms of early cirrhosis include fatigue, decreased appetite and nausea, spots on the skin, and easy bleeding and bruising. Symptoms of late cirrhosis include jaundice, abdominal swelling, leg swelling, confusion, or internal bleeding.

89. What are liver function tests?

Liver function tests are blood tests used to screen for liver disease and to evaluate the liver in patients with known liver disease. A variety of blood tests are available to assess the liver, including tests that analyze inflammation in the liver and tests that analyze the functioning of the liver. Doctors usually order a standard group of tests called a **liver panel** that includes **aspartate aminotransferase (AST)**, **alanine aminotransferase (ALT)**, bilirubin, **alkaline phosphatase**, and albumin. The **aminotransferase** levels reflect the amount of inflammation in the liver, and the albumin and bilirubin levels reflect the functioning of the liver. Alkaline phosphatase levels can rise in many liver conditions, but elevations are especially likely when the bile ducts are blocked.

Liver function tests are blood tests used to screen for liver disease and to evaluate the liver in patients with known liver disease.

Liver panel

Standard group of laboratory tests used to evaluate the functioning of the liver.

AST

See aminotransferases.

Alkaline phosphatase

A blood test that measures injury to the liver or the bile ducts.

ALT

See aminotransferases.

Aminotransferases

Blood tests that measure enzymes found in liver cells. These levels are often elevated in patients with liver disease. AST (aspartate aminotranferase) and ALT (alanine aminotransferase) are the two most commonly measured.

Liver function tests are not perfect. For example, a person can have normal aminotransferase levels and still have inflammation in the liver; similarly, a patient can have normal albumin and bilirubin levels and still have scarring in the liver. Because of this unreliability, your doctor may recommend a liver biopsy to more accurately assess the level of inflammation and scarring. The many different patterns observed with liver function test abnormalities reflect different medical conditions and different levels of functioning in the liver.

Aminotransferase (AST and ALT) levels are used to measure direct injury to liver cells. These enzyme levels are commonly used to screen people for liver disease. They are also used to follow the activity of disease in patients with a known liver disease. These tests are not perfect and your doctor can help you interpret the significance of any changes. There are some liver diseases that are known to often progress even in the setting of normal AST and ALT levels.

As mentioned earlier, the albumin and bilirubin levels taken as part of a standard liver panel reflect the functioning of the liver. Another blood test, called the prothrombin time (PT), reflects the body's ability to clot and is also a good marker of liver function. This test is not in a standard liver profile, however.

The liver produces albumin, which is the main protein in blood. A shortage of albumin can lead to problems with fluid balance and the development of free fluid in the abdomen, a condition known as ascites. The albumin level falls as liver function deteriorates; as a consequence, many doctors follow albumin levels closely in their patients with liver disease. One of the major grading systems for patients with cirrhosis uses the albumin level, bilirubin level, and prothrombin time to judge how well the liver is functioning. Kidney failure and malnutrition are other major reasons that a person might have a low albumin level.

The liver helps break down old red blood cells into bilirubin, which is then excreted into the bile ducts. In liver disease, the bilirubin level may become elevated because the liver is less efficient at clearing and processing old blood cells. As the bilirubin level increases, a person may develop yellow eyes or skin. This condition, which is called jaundice, is a sign of poor liver function. Blockage of the bile duct, blood disorders, and even a benign hereditary condition called Gilbert's syndrome are other reasons that a person might have a high bilirubin level.

Alkaline phosphatase is an enzyme found mostly in the liver and bone. In particular, it is found in the cells that line the bile ducts of the liver. The bile ducts help drain the liver, so any process that blocks bile ducts can lead to an elevation of the alkaline phosphatase level. The most common conditions that lead to such elevations are gallstones in the bile duct, cancers that block the bile duct, strictures of the bile duct, and liver diseases that attack the bile ducts. A very high level should prompt a search for one of the more common conditions that can cause an alkaline phosphatase elevation.

Elevated liver function levels can occur in other medical conditions because the enzymes measured by these tests are present in other parts of the body besides the liver. For example, alkaline phosphatase is found in bone and the placenta and can become elevated in bone disease and pregnancy. Likewise, AST is present in many parts of the body, including muscle, and its level will rise whenever muscle is destroyed, such as during a heart attack. These other conditions need to be considered when the patient does not have obvious liver disease.

90. What types of liver X-rays can be performed?

Blood tests provide a great deal of useful information about the liver but have several limitations, as discussed earlier. To provide even more information about a patient's condition, doctors order a variety of radiological tests that can visualize the liver and other organs in the abdomen, including the gallbladder, kidneys, spleen, pancreas, and blood vessels. The most common imaging test of the liver is the ultrasound. Computed tomography (CT) and magnetic resonance imaging (MRI) scans are typically performed as follow-up measures when the ultrasound shows an abnormality; these tests are discussed later in this question.

The most common imaging test of the liver is the ultrasound.

An ultrasound can provide a lot of information about the liver and the severity of a patient's liver disease. When a patient develops cirrhosis, the size and texture of the liver and spleen may change. Patients who are experiencing liver failure may have a buildup of fluid in the abdomen (called ascites). Patients with cirrhosis are at risk for liver cancer, and an ultrasound can sometimes pick up liver cancer. Ultrasounds are not perfect, however, so they are used in conjunction with other information when assessing a patient's condition.

Your doctor may order an ultrasound for you in many different circumstances. For instance, an ultrasound test may be performed if you have an abnormal liver test. If a person with known liver disease presents with abdominal pain, an ultrasound may be performed to look for abnormalities in the blood vessels that supply the liver. An ultrasound is also useful to guide procedures such as a liver biopsy or a **paracentesis** (a procedure that drains abdominal fluid in patients with ascites).

If you have an ultrasound, this is what you can expect. First, the technician applies a jelly directly to the skin; it will make the images clearer for the doctor reading the test. Next, the technician passes a smooth transducer over the skin. The transducer produces sound waves that go through your skin and bounce against your internal organs. A computer processes this information and produces images that will appear on a screen. An ultrasound is not invasive, painful, or harmful. It can be performed on an outpatient or inpatient basis and takes less than an hour.

CT scans and MRI scans are radiologic tests that can take highly detailed pictures of the liver and other internal organs. These tests are ordered when initial screening tests detect an abnormality or if there is a high degree of clinical concern based on other factors.

A CT scan takes multiple X-rays of the body and uses a computer to generate cross-sectional images—that is, "slices" through the body. CT scans have been around for many years, and most hospitals have a lot of experience with them. A special contrast agent is injected into the patient's vein as the CT scan is being done. This agent helps differentiate blood vessels and can help distinguish hepatomas from benign liver tumors. In a small percentage of patients, the contrast agent may cause an allergic reaction. The contrast agent is also potentially dangerous to the kidneys, so it is generally not used in patients with kidney dysfunction. During the CT scan,

Paracentesis

Procedure where fluid in the abdomen is drained with a needle.

patients are exposed to radiation but the amount per X-ray is relatively low. Repeated CT scans may expose a patient to unnecessary radiation.

MRI scans use radio waves and strong magnets instead of X-rays to create pictures of the body. The radio waves are absorbed by the tissues of the body and released in specific patterns to create a detailed image of the body part that is being examined. A contrast agent is also used when examining the liver. MRI scans may be slightly better at finding liver cancers than CT scans. However, MRI scans are a newer technology, and some hospitals have less experience with them. MRI scans are more uncomfortable than CT scans and can be difficult for patients who are scared of enclosed spaces.

Whether a CT scan or an MRI scan is performed depends on the specific clinical situation, the doctor's preference, and the specific expertise of the radiologists who perform the procedures. Sometimes, both a CT scan and an MRI scan are done in the same patient when the information gathered by one technique is not absolutely clear. Although these tests are clearly superior to an ultrasound, sometimes they may not provide a definitive answer about whether a liver cancer is present. In these cases, the usual approach is to follow the patient closely and repeat the testing in a few months to see if there is any change. A hepatoma would be expected to grow over a few months, whereas a benign tumor would be expected to stay the same size.

91. What is a liver biopsy?

Evaluation with blood tests and radiological tests provides a lot of information, but looking at actual liver tissue is often helpful and necessary to make a medical decision. A liver biopsy is performed in these cases. During a biopsy, a tiny cylinder of tissue is removed; a pathologist then views the sample under a microscope. A liver biopsy can provide critical information about the cause and extent of a patient's liver disease. For example, if a patient presents with abnormal liver tests and a diagnosis is not clear after initial testing, a liver biopsy may be performed to find a diagnosis. A biopsy may help identify causes of liver dysfunction such as a drug reaction, autoimmune hepatitis, alcohol use, or cancer for which blood tests and X-rays are often nonspecific.

A liver biopsy can provide critical information about the cause and extent of a patient's liver disease.

A liver biopsy is usually performed to assess the degree of damage to the liver. If the liver has active inflammation, it can range from mild to severe. Mild disease is characterized by inflammation, but the appearance of liver cells is preserved. As the disease progresses, normal cells are replaced by fibrous tissue. The result may ultimately be cirrhosis, where the liver has scars, nodules (pockets of fibrous tissue), and an irregular appearance.

Many staging systems have been developed for interpreting a liver biopsy. The most widely used system assigns a number between 0 and 4 for the amount of inflammation in the liver (the grade) and a number between 0 and 4 for the amount of scarring in the liver (the stage). Doctors usually focus on the stage (amount of scarring) when deciding on the need for treatment. A stage 0 biopsy is considered normal, whereas a stage 4 biopsy has enough scarring to be classified as cirrhosis. Stages 1, 2, and 3 represent steps between stage 0 and stage 4.

If you have a liver biopsy, this is what you can expect. Your doctor may require you to get blood tests first to ensure that you do not have an increased risk of bleeding after the procedure. In addition, you should discontinue any use of aspirin and aspirin-like products (such as ibu-profen) three to seven days before the biopsy. Ask your doctor about instructions regarding diet. Your doctor may perform the biopsy, or a member of the radiology department may handle the procedure. Initially, your skin will be cleaned with a solution to reduce the risk of infection. Then, the skin is numbed with a medication similar to Novocain used in a dentist's office. Often, a non-invasive device called an ultrasound is used to guide the procedure. A sample of tissue is removed through a needle and sent to the pathology department for further processing. The biopsy may be performed on an inpatient or outpatient basis. Although it takes less than one-half hour, you will be monitored for several hours afterward.

The most common complication of a liver biopsy is pain. This discomfort usually consists of a dull ache in the right-upper abdomen or shoulder and resolves within two hours with or without pain medications. Bleeding, infection, and drug reactions are other less common but potentially serious complications of a biopsy. Unrelenting pain is rare and could indicate a severe complication; notify your doctor immediately if it occurs.

92. What is hepatitis A?

Hepatitis A is a viral infection that can cause hepatitis (inflammation in the liver).

Hepatitis A is transmitted through a "fecal-oral" route. In fecal-oral transmission, the infectious organisms enter the body through ingestion of contaminated food and water. The organisms usually multiply in the digestive system, exit the body through feces, and spread where poor sanitation allows contamination of food or water. Hepatitis A outbreaks, for instance, are commonly traced to food preparers with hepatitis A who have not adequately cleaned their hands. Epidemics are common in low socioeconomic populations where sanitary conditions are less than ideal.

Hepatitis A infection can be asymptomatic, feel like a nonspecific viral infection, or cause an obvious hepatitis picture. Symptoms can include jaundice, fatigue, abdominal pain, loss of appetite, nausea, diarrhea, and fever. In general, symptoms are more common in adults than in children. Many people test positive for immunity to hepatitis A (meaning a previous exposure) but cannot pinpoint when they were exposed. Almost all patients who are infected with hepatitis A recover fully. Hepatitis A never develops into a chronic hepatitis like hepatitis B and hepatitis C often do. Lifelong immunity develops after exposure and you cannot get hepatitis A again. Treatment of acute hepatitis A consists of rest, fluids, and adequate nutrition; hospitalization is rarely required.

Certain groups of people are at higher risk for acquiring hepatitis A. These include household and sexual contacts of infected persons, people living in or traveling to areas of the world where hepatitis A is more common, men who have sex with men, and drug users.

If a person has been or may be exposed to hepatitis A, an immunoglobulin (antibody preparation) can be administered to him or her to prevent infection. This measure provides temporary protection against hepatitis A. The immunoglobulin injection can be given before possible exposure such as a planned trip to a high risk area or within two weeks of a known or suspected exposure.

A vaccination against hepatitis A is also available and provides longer (possibly lifelong) protection. Vaccination should be considered in people 12 months or older who may be at high risk of exposure or increased risk of getting very sick if they develop hepatitis A. These groups include travelers to high risk areas, men who have sex with men, drug users, persons with clotting-factors disorders, persons with chronic liver disease, and children living in areas with increased hepatitis A rates.

93. What is hepatitis B?

Hepatitis B is spread through blood when an uninfected person is exposed to blood from an infected person.

Hepatitis B is a viral infection that can cause both acute and chronic hepatitis. Hepatitis B is spread through blood when an uninfected person is exposed to blood from an infected person. The most common ways of acquiring hepatitis B are through sexual contact, use of IV drugs, and from mother to child during childbirth. About 2 billion people (one third of the world's population) have been exposed to hepatitis B. Many of these people do not develop chronic hepatitis but about 350 to 400 million people are chronically infected and about 1 million people die each year from complications of hepatitis B. If you have chronic hepatitis B, there is a 15 to 25% chance of death from a liver related problem. Most of these people live in areas where hepatitis B is endemic (common) and are exposed to this virus at birth. The United States is not an endemic area for hepatitis B, and less than 2% of the US population has been infected or exposed to hepatitis B. Most cases in the United States are acquired as an adult.

Patients who acquire hepatitis B at birth do not develop acute hepatitis; instead, they typically develop a chronic infection. Chronic infection develops in about 90% of infants infected at birth and 30% of children infected between the ages of one and five years. Patients who are exposed to hepatitis B as adults usually recover completely and rarely develop chronic hepatitis. Symptoms of an acute infection can develop and may include joint pain, rash, fatigue, decreased appetite, nausea, vomiting, and jaundice (yellow skin). Some patients have minimal or nonspecific viral symptoms. About 5–10% of people who are exposed as adults will not clear the virus and will develop chronic hepatitis.

Complications from chronic hepatitis B include cirrhosis, liver failure, and liver cancer. Treatment of acute hepatitis B is similar to treatment of hepatitis A and includes rest, fluids, and adequate nutrition. Treatment of chronic hepatitis is also available; options include **interferon** (shots usually taken for one year) and nucleoside/nucleotide analogs (pills usually taken forever) that interfere with replication of the virus. Patients with chronic hepatitis B are monitored for evidence of active inflammation and liver damage and for liver cancer. Patients with active disease should be considered for treatment and all patients should be screened on a regular basis for liver cancer.

Interferon

Family of proteins naturally produced by the body to fight off infection. There are three types: alfa, beta, and gamma. Alfa interferon is used to treat hepatitis C.

A vaccination for hepatitis B is available and effective in up to 90% of people who receive the **vaccine**. When it was initially developed, the vaccine was given to anyone considered to be at high risk for exposure to hepatitis B or at high risk for a severe infection if exposed. This population included immunocompromised patients, hemodialysis patients, chronic liver disease patients, healthcare workers, injection-drug users, and individuals with high-risk sexual partners. More recently, the vaccine has been used universally and all children are vaccinated after birth. This has led to a dramatic

Vaccine

A preparation of a specific weakened or killed virus or bacterium that is injected to stimulate the immune system.

decrease in new cases of hepatitis B; especially in areas of the world where the infection is common and often transmitted from mother to child at birth.

94. What is hepatitis C?

Hepatitis C is a viral infection that can cause inflammation and scarring in the liver. Hepatitis C rarely causes an acute hepatitis. Most cases are diagnosed by testing patients with risk factors, abnormal liver function tests, or symptoms of chronic hepatitis and cirrhosis. Patients with hepatitis C who progress to cirrhosis can develop complications of liver failure and liver cancer. These complications do not develop in everyone who has hepatitis C. This virus can also affect other parts of the body such as the kidneys and nerves, although complications outside of the liver are very uncommon.

Hepatitis C is spread when blood from an infected person comes into contact with an uninfected person. The most common routes of transmission are blood transfusions and intravenous drug use. Today, significantly fewer new cases of hepatitis C are occurring because blood products are effectively screened for this virus. Instead, most new cases are related to intravenous drug use and the sharing of needles. The number of new infections has declined from about 240,000 per year in the 1980's to about 26,000 in 2004. Other risk factors for acquiring hepatitis C include clotting factors infusions before 1987, blood transfusions before 1992, solid organ transplant before 1992, hemodialysis, and birth to an infected mother. There is a very low risk of infection for people with multiple sex partners, people with a steady sexual partner with a known hepatitis C infection, and healthcare/public safety workers (unless there is a known exposure to infected blood).

Hepatitis C is a very common infection both in the United States and throughout the world. An estimated 170 million people worldwide are infected with this virus. In the United States, almost 4 million people have a positive **antibody** test. Most of these people have chronic hepatitis C and are at risk for developing cirrhosis and subsequent liver failure and liver cancer. Currently, hepatitis C accounts for about 10,000 deaths per year in the United States. This number is expected to increase in the next two decades due to the epidemiology and natural history of this infection. A large number of new infections occurred in the 1960s, 1970s, and 1980s. The peak disease burden from hepatitis C is still ahead of us because progression to cirrhosis can take 20 to 40 years.

Antibody
A protein produced by the body's immune system.

Another way to look at the numbers is by noting that hepatitis C accounts for 15% of cases of acute hepatitis, 60–70% of cases of chronic hepatitis, and 50% of cases of cirrhosis, liver failure, and liver cancer. Roughly half of all liver transplants in the United States now involve patients with hepatitis C. This virus is so common that you probably know at least one person who is infected with it.

Although hepatitis C can have many effects, it primarily attacks the liver. Most people who are exposed to the virus develop a chronic infection. Many people with chronic hepatitis C develop inflammation in the liver, which can in turn lead to scarring. Severe scarring of the liver, which is called cirrhosis, can lead to liver failure and liver cancer. Fortunately, this progression happens in only about 20% of patients with chronic infection. This risk is significantly higher in people who consume excessive amounts of alcohol. Another important point is that patients with cirrhosis do not immediately or even necessarily develop liver failure or liver cancer. Many patients with cirrhosis have an early-stage condition called compensated cirrhosis, in which the liver still functions well and the person can lead a normal life. Patients with HCV-related cirrhosis have a 3 to 4% annual risk of developing liver failure and a 1.4–6.9% annual risk of developing liver cancer. Many of these patients are eligible for liver transplantation. Out of every 100 people exposed to hepatitis C, 55–85 people will develop a chronic infection, 5–20 people will develop cirrhosis, and only 1–5 people will die of cirrhosis and its complications. Hepatitis C occasionally leads to problems outside of the liver, including **cryoglobulinemia**, **glomerulonephritis**, and **porphyria cutanea tarda**.

Anyone with hepatitis C should be careful about spreading the infection to other people. Viruses are spread through a variety of routes, and each virus has different risk factors for its transmission. Hepatitis C is spread through blood-to-blood contact in which HCV-infected blood comes in contact with another person's bloodstream. People with hepatitis C therefore need to be careful about not exposing others to their blood.

Hepatitis C can be spread through sexual activity only if there is blood-to-blood contact. Patients should inform sexual partners of their infection and the risk of transmission. Individuals in monogamous relationships can discuss this issue with their doctors and decide on the appropriate precautions. Patients who are sexually active with multiple partners should always use a new latex condom with lubricants to reduce the risk of bleeding. This practice will protect against the spread of hepatitis C and other infections that can be transmitted sexually. Hepatitis C patients should never donate sperm, ova, or blood.

Cryoglobulinemia

The presence of abnormal proteins in the blood.

Glomerulonephritis

Each kidney is made up of tiny structures called glomeruli that function to produce urine. This type of kidney disease affects the glomeruli through inflammation.

Porphyria cutanea tarda

Blistering skin disease that affects sun exposed areas of the body due to an enzyme deficiency in the liver. It may be precipitated by hepatitis C infection, iron overload, and alcohol use.

Patients should always inform their doctors and dentists about their hepatitis C diagnosis. In addition, health-care workers should routinely wash their hands before and after every patient contact. Needles and other sharp instruments that have been exposed to patient blood are always handled carefully and discarded into special trash receptacles. Although there have been some reported cases involving possible transmission of HCV between patients who have shared instruments or supplies in dental and medical offices, they are very rare.

Blood must be cleaned thoroughly if it spills, because HCV can live for as long as four days on different surfaces. Bloodstains should be cleaned with a bleach solution consisting of 1 part bleach and 10 parts water. At home, do not share razor blades, toothbrushes, nail clippers, or other personal hygiene items with any family members; small amounts of blood on these items may spread infection to others. Always dispose of used feminine hygiene products in plastic bags.

One of the most important questions for patients with hepatitis C is whether treatment is necessary and appropriate.

Hepatitis C is not spread through casual contact so the sharing of cups, plates, and utensils is felt to be safe. Hepatitis C is not spread through hugging and kissing.

One of the most important questions for patients with hepatitis C is whether treatment is necessary and appropriate. This decision is never an emergency and should be considered carefully. Because hepatitis C progresses over years and decades, there is never a medical reason to start treatment urgently. There are many different ways to approach this decision. Some patients have already made a definitive decision by the time of their initial consultation with a gastroenterologist or **hepatologist**.

Hepatologist

A physician whose expertise includes liver diseases and liver transplantation.

Most patients, however, are confused and spend a long time discussing the risks and benefits of treatment. The decision-making process is different for every patient. The medical facts that are discussed here are applicable to everyone. The way that you assess the facts, as well as the way that treatment fits into the rest of your life (with family, work, and friends), is always different and makes each decision making process unique.

Several issues make this a difficult decision to reach. First, most patients with hepatitis C do not progress to cirrhosis and will never develop symptomatic liver disease. Unfortunately, there is no way to predict with absolute certainty who will develop cirrhosis and when that will happen. The best current test is a liver biopsy, but it gives only a snapshot of what the liver currently looks like and is a less than a perfect guide. Therefore, many patients who opt for treatment will probably never progress to cirrhosis even without treatment.

Ribavirin

Synthetic antiviral nucleoside used in the treatment of hepatitis C.

Second, current treatment options all have limitations. Therapy with interferon and **ribavirin** is limited by unwanted side effects and variable cure rates, for example. Many patients are not candidates for treatment, and many patients choose to defer treatment because of these concerns.

Genotype

Because the hepatitis C virus is continually changing or mutating, six major strains of the virus (called genotypes) exist.

Patients who do opt for treatment follow a standardized protocol. They take an interferon shot once a week and ribavirin tablets twice a day. The duration of therapy is determined by the viral **genotype** and the amount of disease found on the initial liver biopsy. The doctor checks the patient's viral levels on a regular basis, and treatment stops if the patient fails to meet predefined goals. Patients are monitored closely for side effects, and treatment is adjusted or stopped as needed. Most studies report overall cure rates of about 50%. We expect newer medicines to be available within the next one to two years.

95. What is hemochromatosis?

Hemochromatosis is a disease characterized by the abnormal accumulation of iron in organs including the liver, pancreas, joints, and heart. Hemochromatosis can result from both genetic and non-genetic causes. Hereditary hemochromatosis is the term used to describe cases resulting from a genetic mutation. Most cases in the United States are due to a specific genetic mutation that is relatively common (about 1 in 200) in high-risk groups such as patients with a Northern European ancestry. More than one million Americans carry this gene mutation. Many, but not all, will develop iron overload, and many of these patients will develop clinical hemochromatosis. Other causes of iron overload include blood disorders, chronic transfusion therapy, excessive iron ingestion, and any type of chronic hepatitis (hepatitis B and hepatitis C are common examples). Chronic hepatitis patients often have elevated iron studies and evidence of iron deposits on liver biopsy but almost never develop significant iron-related liver damage. The level of the iron studies and the location of the iron deposits can help distinguish this nonspecific iron overload from real hemochromatosis. In confusing situations, doctors can order a blood test that looks from the specific gene mutation as discussed below.

This disorder can lead to cirrhosis, diabetes, abnormal skin pigmentation, arthritis, and heart abnormalities. Patients usually remain asymptomatic before the age of 40 because it takes many years for a person to accumulate enough iron to develop organ damage. Early symptoms can include, fatigue, weakness, weight loss, abdominal discomfort, and joint pains. Late liver-related symptoms include all of the standard complications of cirrhosis including liver failure and liver cancer. Other complications of hemochromatosis include heart disease, diabetes, arthritis, bronze skin color, impotence for men, and infertility and premature menopause for women.

Diagnosis can be made through standard blood tests, genetic studies, or liver biopsy depending on the clinical situation. Asymptomatic patients are often diagnosed because of a family history or when blood tests show elevated liver enzymes. Symptomatic patients are diagnosed when they are screened for hemochromatosis because of the development of any of the above symptoms. Genetic studies are usually used to confirm a suspected case. These tests will pick up about 90% of cases of hemochromatosis. A liver biopsy can help identify the other 10% of cases. A liver biopsy is also often used to assess the extent of scarring and damage in the liver. A young patient with classic genetic studies does not necessarily need a liver biopsy because the diagnosis is very certain and the risk of significant damage to the liver is very low.

Hemochromatosis is treated by phlebotomy, which is the same procedure used for blood donors. Phlebotomy works by removing the excess iron in the body because blood contains a large amount of iron. Most people have one to two phlebotomy sessions a week for up to one year to remove the excess iron. Blood tests for iron levels and blood counts are followed closely during this initial treatment phase. Once the iron levels fall to safe levels, the phlebotomy interval is decreased; usually once every two to four months. Blood tests are followed once or twice a year and the frequency of phlebotomy can be adjusted as needed. Patients who are treated before the development of cirrhosis have a great prognosis. Patients who already have cirrhosis need to be monitored closely (as does anyone with cirrhosis) but will have a much lower risk of developing complications after adequate phlebotomy.

Patients diagnosed with hereditary hemochromatosis should inform blood relatives, who should then be screened by their doctors. Parents, grandparents, siblings, and children should be screened. Many patients are diagnosed because of family screening and lives can be saved. Other things to do include avoiding alcohol, avoiding iron supplements (eating iron-containing foods is fine), avoiding excessive vitamin C which helps absorb iron, and avoiding raw fish and shellfish which can contain bacteria dangerous to patients with hemochromatosis.

96. What is fatty liver?

Fatty liver is the lay term used to describe the general condition of having fatty deposits in the liver. The medical term for this condition is **nonalcoholic fatty liver disease (NAFLD)**. NAFLD is divided into two subtypes based on whether there is inflammation and damage in the liver. A liver biopsy is usually necessary to distinguish between the two subtypes. Simple (or benign) fatty liver means that the biopsy shows only fat and no inflammation or scarring. **Nonalcoholic steatohepatitis (NASH)** is the term used to describe the condition of fatty liver with inflammation and scarring. As the name suggests, the biopsy resembles alcoholic liver disease but in people with no history of significant alcohol intake. The distinction is important because patients with NASH are at risk for developing cirrhosis and its complications while patients with benign fatty liver are

Nonalcoholic fatty liver disease (NAFLD)

Liver disease secondary to excessive fatty deposition, usually as a result of obesity.

Nonalcoholic steatohepatitis (NASH)

Liver inflammation caused by buildup of fat in the liver. It occurs in people with no significant alcohol intake.

not. Luckily, most patients with NAFLD have benign fatty liver and not NASH.

The number of patients with NAFLD (fatty liver) in the United States has increased dramatically over the last decade. This increase is probably related to the increasing average weight in this country. Obesity can lead to fatty liver and also contributes to diabetes and high cholesterol, which are also risk factors for fatty liver. However, some patients with NASH are not obese and do not have diabetes or high cholesterol. The prevalence of fatty liver in large studies has varied from 5.5% to 31% depending on the definitions used. Most of these patients have benign fatty liver but some do have NASH and are at risk for developing significant liver disease. The risk for NASH appears to be higher in older patients (age >45–50), and in patients with obesity and diabetes. The exact reason for liver injury is not known but possible theories include insulin resistance, release of cytokines (inflammatory proteins) by fat cells in the liver, and increased oxidation damage (the addition of oxygen to a compound with a loss of electrons) of liver cells.

Fatty liver is usually diagnosed when patients are noted to have abnormal liver function tests often on a routine blood test. Patients usually then have a series of blood tests to exclude other types of liver disease such as hepatitis B, hepatitis C, and hemochromatosis. An ultrasound is often done and can show changes suggestive of fat. The only way to definitively confirm the diagnosis and to distinguish benign fatty liver from NASH is to do a liver biopsy. (Liver biopsy was discussed in **Question 91**) A liver biopsy is not always necessary. A biopsy is usually recommended when there is uncertainty with the diagnosis or concern that there may be more advanced scarring in the liver. In most cases, your doctor will recommend

The number of patients with NAFLD (fatty liver) in the United States has increased dramatically over the last decade.

treating the causes of fatty liver (weight, diabetes, high cholesterol) and following the blood tests closely.

Like many liver diseases, most patients with fatty liver have no symptoms until the development of cirrhosis. Patients with NASH can have a slow progression of scarring in the liver that can take years or even decades to develop cirrhosis. Once a patient with NASH has cirrhosis, he can develop all of the complications seen in anyone with cirrhosis.

There is no specific treatment for NAFLD or NASH. The current recommendations are based on common sense and include weight reduction in obese patients, following a balanced and healthy diet, appropriate physical activity, alcohol avoidance, care with over-the-counter and prescription medications, and treatment of diabetes and high cholesterol if present. Several medicines have been or are being studied in patients with NASH. These studies have looked at two general groups of medicines: antioxidants and antidiabetic medicines. Antioxidants such as vitamin E, selenium, and betaine may help reduce the oxidative damage to liver cells seen in NASH. Newer antidiabetic medicines such as metformin and pioglitazone make the body more sensitive to insulin and may help with the insulin resistance seen in NASH. In severe cases, liver transplantation is necessary and NASH is becoming a major indication for transplant in this country.

97. Are there other types of liver disease?

There are many other types of liver disease but describing all of them in detail is beyond the scope of this book. In this question, I will briefly describe some of the other types of liver disease that are relatively common. Specifically,

I will mention autoimmune hepatitis, primary biliary cirrhosis, and primary sclerosing cholangitis.

Autoimmune hepatitis is a type of hepatitis in which the body's immune system inappropriately attacks liver cells. The immune system functions to protect the body from outside infections such as bacteria and viruses and usually does not attack the body's own cells. Autoimmune diseases can develop when the immune system starts attacking our body's cells. When left untreated over many years, autoimmune hepatitis can lead to cirrhosis and all of the usual complications of cirrhosis. Autoimmune hepatitis is seen more commonly in women (about 70% of cases). Patients often have other autoimmune disorders such as type 1 diabetes, glomerulonephritis (a type of kidney disease), thyroid disease, Sjogren's syndrome (a connective tissue disease), autoimmune anemia, and ulcerative colitis.

Patients with autoimmune hepatitis can present with symptoms or can be found incidentally when abnormal liver function tests are detected. Symptoms depend on the stage of the disease at the time of diagnosis and basically whether cirrhosis has developed or not. Nonspecific symptoms include fatigue, anorexia, nausea, vomiting, abdominal pain, joint pain, rashes, jaundice, dark urine, and light colored stools. Patients with cirrhosis can present with any of the common symptoms of cirrhosis. Autoimmune hepatitis is relatively hard to diagnose because there is no single absolutely reliable blood test like there is with hepatitis B or hepatitis C. Your doctor will probably do a panel of blood tests including special antibody tests and may even recommend a liver biopsy to help confirm the diagnosis. Treatment involves suppressing the immune system. Corticosteroids are usually used initially because they work quickly and are very effective. Patients who require long-term treatment are often transitioned to another medicine called azathioprine. Treatment options vary with each individual case.

Primary biliary cirrhosis (PBC) is a disease that attacks and slowly destroys the small bile ducts in the liver. The exact cause is unknown but this disease may also be an autoimmune disorder. Bile duct destruction eventually leads to cirrhosis after many years. PBC usually affects women between the ages of 30 and 60. PBC is often incidentally diagnosed based on abnormal liver function tests. The most common abnormality is an elevation in the alkaline phosphatase level. The most common symptoms at the time of diagnosis are fatigue and itchy skin. Patients with more advanced disease can present with any of the signs and symptoms of cirrhosis. Patients often have other problems including osteoporosis, arthritis, and thyroid disease. Diagnosis is usually based on blood tests and liver biopsy. A blood test called an antimitochondrial antibody is positive in most patients with PBC. A liver biopsy will show evidence of inflammation and destruction of the small bile ducts. The main medical treatment is a medicine called ursodeoxycholic acid, which is a bile acid that appears to help by increasing bile flow. Vitamin replacement therapy and osteoporosis screening are also important parts of treatment. Ursodeoxycholic acid does not cure PBC but appears to slow down progression of the disease. Liver transplantation is very effective for patients with end stage PBC with decompensated cirrhosis or severe itching.

Primary sclerosing cholangitis (PSC) is related to PBC in that the bile ducts are attacked but in this disease it is the larger bile ducts that are involved. The main complications of PSC include bile duct obstruction, bile duct cancer, and cirrhosis. PSC is often found in patients with ulcerative colitis; which is a type of inflammatory bowel disease. Most patients are men and the usual age of diagnosis is between 30 and 60. The exact cause is unknown with possible theories involving various types of infection or immune system dysfunction. PSC progresses slowly and it usually takes many years before complications develop. The diagnosis is usually suspected because of abnormal blood tests, screening of patients with ulcerative colitis, or symptoms related to bile duct obstruction or cirrhosis. The diagnosis is usually confirmed by taking a picture of the bile ducts with either an MRI scan or by injecting contrast directly into the bile ducts through an endoscopic procedure called an ERCP (endoscopic retrograde cholangiopancreatography). There is no proven effective medical treatment for the underlying disease although patients should be screened for vitamin deficiencies, bone disease, and colon cancer. Patients with bile duct blockage can be treated by endoscopic interventions such as dilatations and stents and occasionally through surgery. Patients with untreatable strictures and with cirrhosis can be treated with liver transplantation. There is no proven effective treatment for patients with bile duct cancers.

98. What is cirrhosis?

The liver is the largest organ in the body and its proper functioning is essential for survival. The liver's many jobs include clearing the blood of toxins, breaking down old red blood cells, creating clotting factors to control bleeding, producing proteins for nutrition, and creating bile to absorb fats and certain vitamins. Cirrhosis is the pathologic condition in which normal liver tissue is replaced by abnormal fibrous scar tissue. This scarring process prevents the liver from functioning properly and makes it harder for blood to flow through the liver.

Because the liver is such an essential organ, its failure creates problems throughout the body. Cirrhosis is the end result of many different chronic liver diseases. The complications associated with its occurrence are the same regardless of the root cause of a patient's liver disease. Cirrhosis kills about 25,000 people per year in the United States, making it the twelfth leading cause of death by disease.

The most common cause of cirrhosis in the United States is excessive consumption of alcohol. Alcoholic cirrhosis often occurs in patients who consume more than four drinks per day for more than 10 years. Approximately 10–15% of people who drink alcohol at this level and for this length of time will develop cirrhosis. Hepatitis C is the second most common cause of cirrhosis in the United States. Up to 20% of patients with hepatitis C develop cirrhosis over a period of 20 to 40 years. Patients who have hepatitis C and drink alcohol have an even higher risk of developing cirrhosis.

Hepatitis B and D are other chronic viral diseases that can progress to cirrhosis. In fact, hepatitis B is the most common cause of cirrhosis worldwide. Autoimmune hepatitis is a disease in which the immune system attacks the liver, producing inflammation and eventually scarring. In addition, several inherited liver diseases can cause cirrhosis. Hemochromatosis is a genetic disorder in which iron is inappropriately stored in various organs. Besides affecting the liver, hemochromatosis can cause fatigue, diabetes, heart failure, arthritis, and various endocrine abnormalities. Other inherited diseases that may cause cirrhosis include alpha-1 antitrypsin deficiency, **Wilson's disease,** and glycogen storage diseases. Finally, chronic diseases of the bile ducts, drugs or toxins, and fatty liver may progress to cirrhosis.

Because the liver is such an essential organ, its failure creates problems throughout the body.

Wilson's disease

A rare inherited disorder in which excessive amounts of copper accumulate in the body. The buildup of copper leads to damage in the kidneys, brain, and eyes.

Because the liver interacts with so many other organs, its failure affects the body in numerous ways. The increased pressure in the liver makes it hard for blood to flow through this organ and leads to a condition called **portal hypertension.** Portal hypertension, in turn, can lead to varices, hemorrhoids, an enlarged spleen, and a low platelet count. The loss of functioning of the liver can also cause ascites, **spontaneous bacterial peritonitis (SBP)**, and **encephalopathy**. Patients with cirrhosis are at an increased risk for developing liver cancer. This risk is higher in certain liver diseases, including viral infections such as hepatitis B and hepatitis C.

A patient with cirrhosis who has not experienced any major complications and still has reasonably good liver function is said to have compensated cirrhosis. Many people with compensated cirrhosis lead normal lives and visit their doctors twice a year for a checkup, blood tests, and an ultrasound to make sure that nothing has changed. Patients with cirrhosis who have had any of the major complications associated with this condition are said to have decompensated cirrhosis. These individuals need active medical care, and many are being evaluated for a liver transplant.

99. What is a liver transplant?

Liver transplantation is a major surgical procedure that involves the removal of a diseased liver and its replacement with a healthy liver. The first successful liver transplant was performed in 1967. Transplant techniques have improved significantly over the last 38 years. In 2005, almost 6,000 adult liver transplants were performed in the United States. Most transplant centers report one year survival rates of at least 85%.

Portal hypertension

Abnormal increase in pressure within the portal system that usually develops in the setting of cirrhosis.

Spontaneous bacterial peritonitis

Infection of ascites that can be treated with antibiotics.

Encephalopathy

See portosystemic encephalopathy (PSE).

The first successful liver transplant was performed in 1967.

A patient with chronic liver disease should be referred for a liver transplant when he or she develops liver failure or liver cancer.

A patient should pursue a transplant when survival is more likely with a transplant than without one. Other reasons for this surgery include congenital birth defects such as **biliary atresia** in children, hereditary diseases where the liver does not properly produce a protein, and benign liver tumors that grow to large sizes and affect the person's quality of life.

Biliary atresia
A blocakge in the tubes (ducts) that carry bile from the liver to the gallbladder.

Transplant centers spend a long time evaluating patients; in fact, this process often takes several months. The evaluation process involves multiple tests of the diseased liver and the patient's general health. Patients also meet with many members of the transplant team, including a hepatologist, transplant surgeon, transplant nurse coordinator, social worker, infectious disease doctor, psychiatrist, financial coordinator, and nutritionist. The transplant team then meets as a group and reviews all of the information gathered during the evaluation. The team assesses the severity of the patient's liver disease, the patient's general health with a focus on his or her ability to survive the surgery, and a psychosocial evaluation. The findings of the transplant committee are discussed at a follow-up appointment and often more tests are required. The decision is often extraordinarily difficult because the current shortage of livers means that not all patients who need a liver transplant will get one. When a person is accepted for transplant, he or she is placed on a list that is currently ordered by disease severity, with the sickest patients appearing at the top of the list. Patients are followed at the transplant center on a regular basis and contacted when a liver becomes available. Unfortunately, sometimes a person becomes too sick to survive a transplant and needs to be taken off of the list.

100. Can prescribed or over-the counter drugs affect the liver?

The liver is involved in the processing of almost all medications. Anyone with liver disease should be careful with new prescription medications and even over-the counter (OTC) medications. Patients without cirrhosis can safely take most—but not all—prescription and OTC medications. Patients with cirrhosis need to be especially careful with their medications. Some common OTC medications, such as acetaminophen (found in Tylenol) and ibuprofen (found in Motrin and Advil), can be very harmful in patients with cirrhosis. Anyone with chronic liver disease should check with his or her doctor before starting any new prescription or OTC medication.

Medications are also a common cause of liver injury and disease and need to be considered whenever anyone presents with a new diagnosis of liver disease. We always take a careful history of all prescription and OTC medications when seeing a patient in initial consultation for a liver problem. In many cases, a reaction to a medication turns out to be the actual cause of the patient's liver disease. More than 900 drugs, toxins, and herbs have been reported to cause liver injury and disease. The range of illness can vary from blood test abnormalities with no symptoms to full blown liver failure. **Fulminant hepatic failure** (FHF) is the term used to describe new onset liver failure in a patient with no preexisting liver disease. Prescription and OTC medications (especially Tylenol) are one of the most common causes of FHF in the United States.

Fulminant hepatic failure (FHF)

The sudden and new onset of liver failure in a patient with no previous liver disease.

A full discussion of drug liver toxicity is beyond the scope of this book. The main points to remember are that patients with chronic liver disease should be careful with all new medications and those patients with new liver problems should have a careful assessment of all medications they are taking or have taken recently.

Glossary

A

Abdominal X-ray: A radiological examination that provides an image of structures and organs in the abdomen-helpful in detecting a bowel obstruction or perforation.

Abscess: A walled-off collection of pus; in Crohn's disease an abscess is most commonly found around the anus or rectum, but can occur anywhere in the body.

Acute: Sudden or severe onset.

Acute pancreatitis: Sudden inflammation of the pancreas, most often caused by alcohol or gallstones. Acute pancreatitis generally causes severe pain in the upper abdomen as well as nausea and vomiting.

Adenocarcinoma: A certain type of cancer characterized by the presence of glands when examined under the microscope. This is the kind of cancer associated with Barrett's esophagus.

Achalasia: A motility disorder of the esophagus producing symptoms of difficulty swallowing.

Adhesions: Formation of scar tissue, usually occurring after surgery, which can produce a blockage.

Albumin: A protein produced by the liver that accounts for most of the protein in blood.

Alkaline phosphatase: A blood test that measures injury to the liver or the bile ducts.

Alpha-fetoprotein (AFP): A blood test that is often elevated in patients who have liver cancer.

ALT: See aminotransferases.

Aminosalicylate: A class of drugs used in Crohn's disease and ulcerative colitis. Also known as 5-ASA.

Aminotransferases: Blood tests that measure enzymes found in liver cells. These levels are often elevated in patients with liver disease. AST (aspartate aminotranferase) and ALT (alanine aminotransferase) are the two most commonly measured.

Ampulla of Vater: Opening of the small intestine where the bile duct and pancreatic duct join and drain into the small intestine.

Amylase: Enzyme produced by the pancreas which plays a role in the digestion of starch. Because levels of amylase in the bloodstream are increased in acute pancreatitis, checking a blood test for amylase is an important tool for diagnosing this disorder.

Anemia: A term used to refer to a low red blood cell count.

Anoscopy: A procedure in which a rigid, short, straight, lighted tube is used to examine the anal canal; usually performed on a special tilt table that positions the patient with the head down and butt up-excellent test to examine for an anal fissure or hemorrhoids.

Antacid: A medication available over the counter, effective for active symptoms of reflux. Antacids work by neutralizing acid on contact. Many types are available without a doctor's prescription.

Antibody: A protein produced by the body's immune system to fight disease.

Antineutrophil cytoplasmic antibody (ANCA): An antibody found in the blood that is associated with the presence of ulcerative colitis.

Antioxidant: Vitamins, minerals, and enzymes that reduce damage to cells by neutralizing free radicals.

Anti-Saccharomyces cerevisiae antibody (ASCA): An antibody found in the blood that is associated with the presence of Crohn's disease.

Anus: The outside opening of the rectum.

Arthritis: Inflammation of the joints; individuals with arthritis often have pain, redness, tenderness, and swelling in the affected joints.

Ascites: Abnormal fluid accumulation in the abdomen that can develop when the liver does not function properly.

AST: See aminotransferases.

Autoimmune: An inflammatory process in which our immune system attacks part of our own body, such as the colon in ulcerative colitis.

Autoimmune hepatitis: A liver disease characterized by an overactive immune system that attacks the liver.

B

Bacterial overgrowth: A condition in which there is an overgrowth of normal intestinal flora; usually seen in the setting of an intestinal stricture.

Barium enema: A radiologic examination of the rectum and colon performed by instilling barium through the rectum and taking X-rays as it goes through the colon-excellent test to detect strictures, inflammation, and fistulas in the colon.

Barrett's esophagus: An inflammatory condition of the esophagus caused by chronic gastroesophageal reflux disease. Barrett's esophagus is a more acid-resistant lining of the esophagus that can predispose a person to the development of esophageal cancer.

Benign: A non-cancerous growth.

Biliary atresia: A blocakge in the tubes (ducts) that carry bile from the liver to the gallbladder.

Bile: Thick, green fluid produced by the liver which plays an important role in the digestion of fats. Bile is made by the liver, stored by the gallbladder, and released into the bile duct and small intestine after meals.

Bile duct: Tube connecting the liver and small intestine. Bile is produced by the liver and flows through the bile duct into the small intestine.

Bilirubin: Product of the breakdown of hemoglobin, which can be measured to evaluate the liver and gallbladder.

Biopsy: The removal of a small piece of tissue.

Body mass index (BMI): Measure of body fat calculated directly from height and weight; used as a screening tool to identify weight problems in adults.

Bowel: Term used for both the large and small intestines.

C

Cancer: An uncontrolled growth of cells in the body that can spread, or metastasize, to other areas of the body.

Capsule endoscopy: Procedure in which a tiny camera is ingested to investigate the esophagus and small bowel.

Cataracts: A clouding of the eyes' natural lens; occurs naturally with age, but the development can be accelerated with chronic use of corticosteroids.

Cell: The smallest unit in the body; millions of cells attached together make up our organs and tissues.

Celiac disease: Hereditary disorder that involves intolerance to gluten, a protein found in wheat, barley and rye.

Centers for Disease Control (CDC): The federal facility for disease eradication, epidemiology, and education that is located in Atlanta, Georgia.

Cholangitis: An inflammation of the bile ducts caused by bacteria.

Cholecystectomy: Surgical removal of the gallbladder. The preferred technique is called laparoscopic cholecystectomy. The surgeon removes the gallbladder by inserting instruments into four small incisions in the abdominal wall. The traditional technique, sometimes called "open cholecystectomy," requires a larger incision in the right upper abdomen. Because of this larger scar, the pain after surgery and overall recovery time are longer with open cholecystectomy.

Cholecystostomy: Drainage tube placed from the skin directly into the gallbladder. This tube is placed to treat infection of the gallbladder called acute cholecystitis. Cholecystotomy tubes are placed when patients are too ill to withstand surgery to remove the gallbladder.

Chronic: Usually refers to a disease that develops slowly and lasts for a long time.

Chronic pancreatitis: Ongoing inflammation of the pancreas, most often caused by alcohol, although in many cases the cause is unknown. Symptoms of this disorder include chronic abdominal pain, nausea and vomiting, loose stools due to impaired digestion of nutrients called steatorrhea, weight loss, and diabetes due to destruction of the cells in the pancreas that produce insulin.

Crohn's disease: A chronic inflammatory disease, primarily involving the small and large intestine, but which can affect other parts of the digestive system as well. Abdominal pain, diarrhea, vomiting, fever, and weight loss are common symptoms.

Chymotrypsin: Enzyme produced by the pancreas which is important in the digestion of proteins.

Cirrhosis: Formation of permanent scar tissue in the liver due to a chronic condition.

Clostridium difficile (*C. diff.*): this is an unhealthy bacterium that can overpopulate the colon, usually as a result of antibiotic use, and lead to colitis symptoms with diarrhea and cramps. It is treated by the antibiotics Flagyl or Vancomycin

Collagenous colitis: A type of microscopic colitis that involves inflammation of the colon and can lead to symptoms of watery diarrhea.

Colitis: inflammation of the colon; can be due to Crohn's disease, ulcerative colitis, or other diseases.

Colon: Large intestine that processes and stores waste.

Colonoscopy: An instrument inserted into the rectum to examine the colon. A long, thin camera with a light source that can be steered once inserted and can enable the physician to take pictures, perform biopsies, or remove polyps.

Constipation: Having fewer than three bowel movements per week. It can also be defined as having hard stools or straining to have a bowel movement.

Contamination: The process of rendering impure or unsuitable by contact; mixture or introduction of an undesirable element.

Corticosteroid: A potent anti-inflammatory drug.

Crohn's disease: A chronic inflammatory disease, primarily involving the small and large intestine, but, which can affect other parts of the digestive system as well.

Cryoglobulinemia: The presence of abnormal proteins in the blood.

CT (computed tomography) Scan: Type of X-ray examination which records images of the internal organs. This exam generally requires the patient to drink a milky white contrast agent beforehand. In addition, intravenous contrast is often given to enhance the quality of the images. This exam is particularly useful for examination of the pancreas in acute pancreatitis.

Cystic fibrosis (CF): Inherited chronic disease that affects the lungs and digestive system due to a defective gene that results in the body to produce unusually thick, sticky mucus.

D

Dehydration: Reduction of water content.

Deooxynucleic acid (DNA): A material inside cells that contains the genetic code for each specific individual.

Diabetes: Elevated blood sugar (glucose).

Distention: Abdominal bloating, usually from excess amounts of gas in the intestines; can be a sign of a bowel obstruction.

Diverticulitis: An infection of a Diverticulum. This infection can cause a "micro" perforation or tiny hole in the colon wall and create a pocket of pus or abscess.

Diverticulosis: Outpouchings in the lining of the colon. When these become inflamed, they can produce symptoms of abdominal pain and fever.

Duodenum: The first part of the small intestine starting at the end of the stomach.

Dysphagia: Difficulty swallowing; the sensation during swallowing of food getting stuck somewhere in the neck or chest.

Dysplasia: A pre-malignant cellular change seen on biopsy prior to the development of cancer; can occur in the colon in ulcerative colitis or Crohn's colitis, but can also be found in other organs not related to IBD, such as cervical dysplasia (which is what a pap smear examines for) or esophageal dysplasia in Barrett's esophagus.

E

Edema: Excess fluid in the body that can cause swelling of extremities and abdomen.

Encephalopathy: See portosystemic encephalopathy (PSE).

Endoscope: Thin, flexible tube with an attached light that is used to view the digestive tract.

Endoscopic Ultrasound (EUS): An instrument similar to endoscopes but also has the capabilities to perform ultrasound. Ultrasound allows investigation of the wall of the lining of the gastrointestinal tract and beyond.

Enteroclysis: A radiologic examination that provides a detailed examination of the small bowel. A small tube is passed through the nose, into the stomach, and out into the duodenum; barium is then instilled through the tube and directly into the small bowel-excellent test to detect small abnormalities in the small intestine that may not have been seen on a small bowel follow through.

ERCP (endoscopic retrograde cholangiopancreatography): Procedure combining endoscopy and X-ray to evaluate the bile duct and pancreatic duct. The most common reason for performing an ERCP is the suspicion of a gallstone stuck in the bile duct.

Esophagitis: Inflammation of the lining of the esophagus that is present in about half of those with chronic reflux symptoms. Esophagitis is diagnosed either by performing a barium study or by endoscopy. Symptoms of esophagitis are heartburn and occasional difficulty swallowing, and it is treated with proton pump inhibitors or H2 blockers.

Esophagus: Tube that carries food from the mouth to the stomach.

Extracorporeal shock wave lithotripsy (ESWL): Noninvasive technique using high-energy sound waves to break up gallstones. Because this procedure is most frequently performed to break up kidney stones, it is generally performed by a urologist.

Extraintestinal manifestations: Signs of IBD that are found outside of the gastrointestinal tract, hence the term "extraintestinal."

F

FDA (Food and Drug Administration): the federal agency that is primarily responsible for overseeing the nations drug approval process, and for monitoring drug safety.

Fiber: A substance in foods that comes from plants. Fiber helps with digestion by keeping stool soft so that it moves smoothly through the colon.

Fissure: A crack or split which, in IBD, is most often seen in the anal canal.

Fistula: A tunnel connecting two structures that are not normally connected; examples include a fistula between the rectum and vagina (rectovaginal fistula), or the colon and bladder (colovesicular fistula).

Food allergy: Reaction of the immune system to something eaten that may result in tingling in the mouth, swelling of the throat, hives, abdominal pain, vomiting, or diarrhea.

Food intolerance: An adverse reaction to food that does not involve the immune system.

Fulminant hepatic failure (FHF): The sudden and new onset of liver failure in a patient with no previous liver disease.

G

Gallbladder: Pouch connected to the bile ducts that stores bile which is released with eating to aid in digestion.

Gallstones: Particles ranging in size from fine specks to firm concretions one inch in diameter. Although gallstones are silent in most individuals, in about 20% of people they cause problems either by inflaming the gallbladder, blocking flow out of the bile duct, or obstructing drainage of the pancreas.

Gastroenteritis: An intestinal illness characterized by abdominal cramps and diarrhea; usually caused by an infection.

Gastroenterologist: A physician who specializes in diseases of the gastrointestinal tract, liver, and pancreas.

Gastrointestinal tract: The digestive tube starting at the mouth and ending at the anus.

General Anesthesia: A form of deep sedation in which patients are given medicines to induce a state of unresponsiveness; patients under general anesthesia will not feel even painful stimuli.

Genotype: Because the hepatitis C virus is continually changing or mutating, six major strains of the virus (called genotypes) exist. .

GERD: Gastroesophageal reflux disease. A disease made up of symptoms of heartburn, reflux, and/or regurgitation.

Glomerulonephritis: Each kidney is made up of tiny structures called glomeruli that function to produce urine. This type of kidney disease affects the glomeruli through inflammation.

Glucagon: Hormone produced by specialized cells in the pancreas called islet cells. Release of glucagon into the bloodstream causes blood sugar levels to increase.

Granuloma: A certain type of cell found in Crohn's disease; can also be seen in other, non-gastrointestinal diseases.

H

H2 blocker: A drug that generally does not require a prescription and is available over the counter. These drugs decrease acid production by the stomach. H2 blockers are effective for esophagitis, GERD, and peptic ulcer disease. They are best used to prevent GERD symptoms and are safe for long-term use. Examples are ranitidine (Zantac), famotidine (Pepcid), nizitadine (Axid), and cimetidine (Tagamet).

Heartburn: The sensation of burning discomfort or warmth traveling up from the stomach into the chest. A symptom of GERD.

Helicobacter pylori (*H. pylori*): A bacterium that lives in the stomach and can cause stomach ulcers. It is diagnosed usually by biopsy of the stomach and treated with 10 to 14 days of antibiotics and antacid medication.

HELLP syndrome (Hemolysis, Elevated **L**iver Enzymes and **L**ow **P**latelets**):** Life threatening condition occurring during the later stages of pregnancy.

Hemorrhoids: Inflammation of the blood vessels around the anus or lower rectum.

Hepatic: A term used to refer to anything pertaining to the liver.

Hepatitis: Inflammation of the liver that causes cell damage.

Hepatocellular carcinoma: See hepatoma.

217

Hepatologist: A physician whose expertise includes liver diseases and liver transplantation.

Hepatoma (HCC): Primary cancer of the liver that often occurs in the setting of cirrhosis.

Hiatal hernia or hiatus hernia: This is the condition where a small or large portion of the stomach, which is usually in the abdomen, pushes through a hole in the diaphragm into the chest. This is often associated with heartburn and GERD.

Hyperemesis gravidarum: Severe nausea and vomiting typically occurring during the beginning stages of pregnancy.

Hypertension: High blood pressure.

I

Immune dysregulation: Failure of the body to appropriately regulate the immune system; this lack or regulation is believed to be integral to the development of Crohn's disease and ulcerative colitis, as well as autoimmune hepatitis.

Immune system: An internal network of organs, cells, and structures that work to guard us against foreign substances, such as infections.

Induction of remission: Use of drug therapy to treat active symptoms and bring about a remission.

Inflammation: A process characterized by swelling, warmth, redness, and/or tenderness; can occur in any organ.

Inflammatory bowel disease (IBD): A group of inflammatory conditions of the large intestine and, in some cases, the small intestine.

Insulin: Hormone produced by specialized cells in the pancreas called islet cells. Insulin has a vital role in the metabolism of sugar-release of insulin into the bloodstream causes blood sugar levels to decrease. Absence of insulin leads to diabetes. Patients with severe chronic pancreatitis can no longer make insulin and therefore become diabetic.

Interferon: Family of proteins naturally produced by the body to fight off infection. There are three types: alfa, beta, and gamma. Alfa interferon is used to treat hepatitis C.

Intrahepatic cholestasis of pregnancy: Itching and yellowing of the skin usually occurring during the late stages of pregnancy.

Irritable bowel syndrome (IBS): Symptoms of diarrhea in the absense of disease pathology.

Ischemic colitis: A medical condition in which inflammation and injury of the colon/large intestine result from inadequate blood supply.

Islet cells: Specialized cells in the pancreas which produce insulin and glucagon, which control the levels of sugar in the bloodstream.

J

Jaundice: Yellowing of the skin due to buildup of bile. The most common causes of jaundice are hepatitis (infection of the liver), and blockage of the outflow of bile from the liver into the intestine from either a stone in the bile duct or a tumor.

K

Kidney stones: Stones that form in the kidneys.

Kwashiorkor: Malnutrition from inadequate protein intake often resulting in generalized swelling, loss of muscle, and increased susceptibility to infections.

L

Lactose intolerance: Common disorder caused by lack of a digestive enzyme that normally breaks down sugars found in milk resulting in diarrhea, cramps, and gas.

Large intestine: See colon.

Latent tuberculosis: A tuberculosis infection that is dormant (inactive infection).

Laxative: Something that loosens the bowels. Used to combat constipation (and sometimes overused, producing diarrhea). The word "laxative" comes from the Latin "laxare" meaning "to open, widen, extend, release."

Left-sided colitis: Ulcerative colitis involving the left side of the colon.

Lipase: Enzyme produced by the pancreas which plays a role in digestion of fats. Because levels of lipase in the bloodstream are increased in acute pancreatitis, checking a blood test for lipase is an important tool for diagnosing acute pancreatitis. In acute pancreatitis, levels of lipase peak in the bloodstream later than amylase.

Liver: Solid organ of the alimentary tract involved in breakdown of toxins and formation of proteins

Liver Biopsy: A test where a small needle is passed into the liver and a piece of the liver is removed and examined under a microscope.

Liver Panel: Standard group of laboratory tests used to evaluate the functioning of the liver. Tests usually include aspartate aminotransferase (AST), alanine aminotransferase (ALT), alkaline phosphatase, albumin, and bilirubin.

Liver Transplant: A major surgical procedure that involves the removal of a diseased liver and the insertion of a healthy liver.

Lower esophageal sphincter (LES): A circular muscle at the bottom of the esophagus above the stomach. This muscle opens when food enters the esophagus, allowing the food passage into the stomach, and contracts, or closes, in between swallows. This muscle, or sphincter, may be too loose or may open at inappropriate times, allowing material to reflux from the stomach up into the esophagus.

Lymphoma: Cancer of the lymphatic system; i.e., lymph nodes.

Lymphocyte: A type of inflammatory cell. Lymphocytes can be normally found in the blood, tissues, and organs throughout the body.

Lymphocytic colitis: A type of microscopic colitis that involves inflammation of the colon and can lead to symptoms of watery diarrhea.

M

Maintenance of remission: The term used to describe the use of drug therapy to maintain a patient in remission.

Malabsorption: A condition in which the small intestine is not able to absorb nutrients and vitamins.

Malignancy: Another term for cancer.

Malnutrition: Insufficient nutrients to maintain healthy bodily functions.

Marasmus: Malnutrition from inadequate protein and caloric intake.

Microbe: A very tiny organism.

Microscopic colitis: A form of inflammatory bowel disease that can be found in the colon. Microscopic colitis causes non-bloody diarrhea. The inflammation

can only be seen under a microscope and not with the naked eye, hence the term "microscopic."

MRI: A type of X-ray exam which uses magnetic energy. MRI is useful for evaluating the solid organs of the abdominal cavity such as the liver and pancreas. MRI is particularly helpful in evaluating the main tube of the pancreas called the pancreatic duct, which can be diseased in chronic pancreatitis.

Mucosa: Inside lining of the intestinal tract.

N

Nasogastric tube: A long, flexible tube that passes through the nose into the stomach; this tube is used to suction out the stomach in the setting of a bowel obstruction, or sometimes after an operation.

Nonalcoholic fatty liver disease (NAFLD): Liver disease secondary to excessive fatty deposition, usually as a result of obesity.

Nonalcoholic steatohepatitis (NASH): Liver inflammation caused by buildup of fat in the liver. It occurs in people with no significant alcohol intake.

Nonsteroidal anti-inflammatory drugs (NSAIDs): A class of medication generally used to treat pain. All NSAIDs can cause irritation or ulcers of the gastrointestinal tract. Examples are aspirin, ibuprofen (Motrin, Advil), and naproxen (Aleve).

O

Obstruction: A blockage; can be in any portion of the intestinal tract or bile ducts.

Osteonecrosis: Also called avascular necrosis, severe deterioration of the bone; it can be seen after long-term use of corticosteroids and is usually diagnosed by an MRI of the affected joint.

Osteoporosis: A severe decrease in bone density; can be seen after long-term use of corticosteroids.

P

Pancolitis: Extensive ulcerative colitis; ulcerative colitis that extends beyond the left colon.

Pancreas: Oblong organ in the upper abdomen with two distinct functions: (1) Enzymes produced by the pancreas are critical for the digestion of food, and (2) Specialized cells in the pancreas called islet cells make insulin and glucagons, which control the levels of sugar in the bloodstream.

Paracentesis: Procedure where fluid in the abdomen is drained with a needle.

Pathologist: A physician trained in the evaluation of organs, tissues, and cells, usually under a microscope; assists in determining and characterizing the presence of disease.

Perforation: A rupture or abnormal opening of the intestine; allows intestinal contents to escape into the abdominal cavity.

Perianal: The adjacent area around the outside of the anus; common site for abscess and fistula formation.

Peristalsis: Movement of the muscles that line the intestinal tract.

Peritonitis: Inflammation of the lining that surrounds organs in the abdominal cavity.

Pharynx: Structure in the throat that connects directly with the beginning of the intestinal tract or esophagus.

Polyps: Growths of the lining of the colon that are benign or premalignant. Adenomas are polyps that have the potential to develop into a cancer if left in place for 10 to 15 years. Hyperplastic polyps are benign polyps.

Porphyria cutanea tarda: Blistering skin disease that affects sun exposed areas of the body due to an enzyme deficiency in the liver. It may be precipitated by hepatitis C infection, iron overload, and alcohol use.

Portal hypertension: Abnormal increase in pressure within the portal system that usually develops in the setting of cirrhosis.

Primary Sclerosing Cholangitis (PSC): Inflammation and scarring of the bile ducts within the liver; can be seen in IBD.

Proctitis: Inflammation of the rectum.

Proctoscopy: A procedure in which a rigid, straight, lighted tube is used to examine the rectum; usually on a special tilt table that positions the patient with the head down and butt up. While this procedure has mostly been replaced by flexible sigmoidoscopy, this is still an excellent test to examine the rectum.

Proton pump inhibitor (PPI): A drug that blocks acid production by the stomach; believed to be stronger and more effective than H2 blockers are. The most effective medicine available to treat acid damage to the esophagus and GERD. Generally recommended for those with severe GERD, esophageal strictures, or Barrett's esophagus. An over-the-counter example is Prilosec. Prescription examples are omeprazole, esomeprazole (Nexium), pantoprazole (Protonix), and lansoprazole (Prevacid).

Pseudocyst: Fluid-filled collection of tissue in or adjacent to the pancreas. Pseudocysts form as a consequence of either acute or chronic pancreatitis and can cause problems when they become infected or grow so large that they block digestion of nutrients or drainage of pancreas juice.

R

Rectum: Last part of the colon where stool is stored before it leaves digestive tract.

Recurrence: The reappearance of a disease.

Reflux: The movement of food, fluid, or acid up from the stomach into the esophagus.

Remission: The state of having no active disease; can refer to clinical remission, meaning no symptoms; endoscopic remission, meaning no disease seen endoscopically; histologic remission, meaning no active inflammation on biopsy.

Rheumatoid arthritis: A type of chronic joint inflammation.

Ribavirin: Synthetic antiviral nucleoside used in the treatment of hepatitis C.

Risk: The chance or probability that something will or will not happen.

Risk factor: Things that predispose someone for getting a disease; as example, smoking is a risk factor for lung cancer.

S

Salivary gland: Glands in the mouth that produce material that aid in the breakdown of food.

Scleroderma: An autoimmune condition that can affect any part of the body and is characterized by thickening and scarring of affected organs.

Secretin test: A test to measure how well the pancreas is functioning. Because the test is somewhat invasive (it requires a nasogastric tube) and cumbersome, it is only performed in specialized centers.

Sedation: Also called conscious sedation, or moderate sedation; sedation is a form of moderate anesthesia in which the patient is given medication to induce a state of relaxation; patients under sedation are sleepy and are less likely to feel discomfort.

Short bowel syndrome: Condition due to loss of a significant amount of small intestine from surgery or certain diseases causing malnourishment from inadequate absorption.

Side effect: An adverse reaction to a medication or treatment.

Sigmoidoscopy: This procedure is basically a "short" colonoscopy and is used to examine the rectum and left colon.

Sign: Objective evidence of disease; something that can be identified on physical examination or by a test.

Small bowel bacterial overgrowth: Abnormally large number of bacteria present in the small intestine that can lead to gas, bloating, diarrhea, and vitamin deficiencies.

Small intestine: The small bowel is made up of the duodenum, jejunum, and ileum. Anatomically it is found after the stomach and before the colon and is responsible for digestion and absorption of nutrients.

Spontaneous Bacterial Peritonitis: Infection of ascites that can be treated with antibiotics.

Squamous cell carcinoma: A type of cancer that can occur in many areas. The commonly seen cancer in the head and neck or esophagus associated with smoking. Under the microscope, there are no glands. Squamous cell carcinoma can occur in the esophagus, but adenocarcinoma is associated with Barrett's esophagus.

Steatorrhea: Loose, oily stools containing fat. Steatorrhea occurs in chronic pancreatitis, when the pancreas is so damaged that it no longer produces enough enzymes to digest fats effectively.

Stent: Tube composed of either plastic or metal which is used to bypass a blockage in the body. In particular, a stent is placed in the bile duct to bypass a narrowing in the bile duct from either benign inflammation or tumor. The bile then flows through the stent from the liver into the small intestine, which preserves the role of bile in digestion and prevents infection that can result from complete blockage of the duct.

Steroid: Another name for corticosteroid; a potent anti-inflammatory drug.

Steroid-dependent: An individual who responds to a corticosteroid, but has a flare upon tapering.

Steroid-refractory: An individual who does not have symptomatic improvement with a corticosteroid.

Stomach: Organ that mixes and breaks down food particles.

Stricture: A narrowed area of intestine usually due to scar tissue.

Symptom: Subjective evidence for disease; something that the patient feels.

Systemic: A process that involves the whole body, as opposed to a localized process; for example, fatigue is a systemic symptom, whereas lower back pain is a local symptom.

T

Tagged red blood cell scan: Also called a bleeding scan; a radiologic procedure done on patients who are actively bleeding internally, but the exact location of the bleeding is unclear. This test involves injection into the bloodstream of radioactively "tagged" red blood cells. A nuclear scan of the body is then performed to better determine the general location of the bleeding. This test is often ordered in patients who have diverticular bleeding, to determine where in the colon this bleeding is happening.

Tenesmus: Intense rectal spasm, usually due to inflammation.

TNF: Tumor necrosis factor; this protein plays a central role in the initiation of inflammation in IBD; first described in the setting of tumors, we now know that TNF is commonly found in many inflammatory conditions.

Topical therapy: A type of therapy that is applied directly to tissue; commonly used in inflammation of the rectum and left colon.

Total parenteral nutrition (TPN): Nutrition solution containing salts, sugars, and fats that is given intravenously for patients who cannot eat or cannot absorb enough nutrients by eating.

TPMT: Thiopurine methyltransferase; one of the body's enzymes responsible for breaking down the drugs azathioprine (Imuran) and 6-MP. A blood test to check a TPMT level is generally drawn prior to initiation of one of these drugs. This is because a small percentage of the population lacks this enzyme and has a higher risk of side-effects.

Transit study: A study to evaluate the function of the colon using small capsules that can be seen on X-ray.

Trypsin: Enzyme produced by the pancreas which is important in the digestion of proteins.

Tuberculosis: An infection with Mycobacterium tuberculosis.

Tumor: An abnormal growth of tissue; can be benign or malignant.

U

Ulcer: An area of damage or a break in the lining of the gut. An ulcer can occur anywhere in the gastrointestinal tract. Classically, ulcers occur in the stomach or duodenum.

Ulcerative colitis: A relatively common disease that causes inflammation of the large intestine (the colon). The cause is unknown. It is a form of inflammatory bowel disease. It has some similarity to a related disorder, Crohn's disease.

Ultrasound: Noninvasive form of X-ray imaging using sound waves. Ultrasound is particularly good at detecting gallstones in the gallbladder.

Upper Endoscopy: see EGD.

Upper GI series/Upper GI series with small bowel follow through: A radiologic examination of the esophagus, stomach, duodenum, and small bowel; performed by having the patient drink a thick, white liquid shake of barium, and taking X-rays as it goes through the gastrointestinal tract-excellent test to detect strictures, fistulas, and inflammation in the stomach and small bowel.

Urgency: The feeling that one has to move their bowels or urinate right away.

V

Vaccine: A preparation of a specific weakened or killed virus or bacterium that is injected to stimulate the immune system.

Varices: Abnormal blood vessels that can form in the esophagus and stomach in a patient with liver disease that can lead to gastrointestinal bleeding.

Villi: Finder like projections lining the small intestine involved in digestion and absorption of food and nutrients.

Virtual colonoscopy: A CT scan of the colon; this radiological study is still in early development but shows promise as a method to detect colonic abnormalities.

W

Whipple's disease: Rare disorder of middle-aged men in which a bacteria damages the small intestine to result in malabsorption, resulting in fever, arthritis, skin changes, and dementia.

Wilson's disease: A rare inherited disorder in which excessive amounts of copper accumulate in the body. THe buildup of copper leads to damage in the kidneys, brain, and eyes.

X

X-ray: A radiologic study that provides an image of bodily structures.

Index

Vitamin K, bilirubin and, 21
Vitamins, 92
    antioxidant, 153

W

Water supply, travelers' diarrhea and, 125
Weight loss
    celiac disease and, 98, 99
    colon cancer and, 133
    Crohn's disease and, 44, 48
    gastrointestinal-related causes of,
        14–15
    malabsorption and, 96
    ulcers and, 31
Weight management, gastroesophageal
    disease and, 39
Whipple's disease, 94
Wilson's disease, cirrhosis of the liver and, 205
Women
    cholesterol stones and, 171
    constipation and, 7
    irritable bowel syndrome and, 18
    microscopic colitis and, 81
World Health Organization, 180

X

X-rays
    of the liver, 184–186
    of the pancreas, 166
    testing for parasites and, 129

Z

Zantac (ranitidine), 34, 39
Zelnorm (tegaserod), ischemic colitis and,
    83
Zollinger-Ellison Syndrome, 15